The Butterfly Caste

The Butterfly Caste

A Social History of
Pellagra in the
South

Elizabeth W. Etheridge

Contributions in
American History, Number 17

Greenwood Publishing Company
Westport, Connecticut

For
Professor Horace Montgomery

Library of Congress Cataloging in Publication Data

Etheridge, Elizabeth W
The butterfly caste.

(Contributions in American history, no. 17)
Bibliography: p.
1. Pellagra--history. 2. Southern States--Social
conditions. 3. Malnutrition. I. Title.
RA645.P4E8   614.5'93'930975   70-176431
ISBN 0-8371-6276-9

Library of Congress Catalog Card Number: 70-176431
ISBN: 0-8371-6276-9

First published in 1972

Greenwood Publishing Company
A Division of Greenwood Press, Inc.
51 Riverside Avenue, Westport, Connecticut 06880

Printed in the United States of America

Contents

List of
Illustrations

Preface

PELLAGRA, SCOURGE OF southern Europe for almost two hundred years, appeared somewhat mysteriously in the American South in the early years of the twentieth century, spread rapidly for no apparent reason, and left panic in its wake. It took a heavy toll of American lives, sent many people to insane asylums (as they were then called), and left others ostracized by their friends and neighbors and even by their own families. The characteristic mark of a pellagrin was a skin rash that symmetrically marked the hands and feet and sketched an ugly red butterfly across the victim's face. This mark of the butterfly became a stigma, which set pellagrins in a caste apart. Some were even isolated as lepers.

At first, this stigma applied only to the unfortunate pellagrins themselves, who were almost invariably poor. Middle and upper classes were spared. But, as the years passed and pellagra began to shed its mystery, it became closely identified with the poverty of the region, and the stigma of the butterfly caste was transferred from individuals to the South as a whole. "The land of hookworm and pellagra," the northern press dubbed the region. Proud Southerners were furious. They eagerly sought cases in other sections of the nation and gloated over every find. When, in 1921, President Warren G. Harding launched an effort to wipe out the disease, angry Southerners accused him of slurring the South, and they denied, not too convincingly, that pellagra even existed.

The puzzle of pellagra was unraveled in large part by Dr. Joseph Goldberger of the United States Public Health Service in the years after 1914. Until he began his work, there was a frantic effort on the part of Southern physicians to find the cause of and a cure for the disease. They blamed it variously on eating corn, spoiled and unspoiled, on the buffalo gnat, housefly, or mosquito and attempted to treat it with everything from arsenic compounds to electric shock. When Goldberger traced the disease to the then new idea of a nutritional shortage, Southern physicians would not accept his findings.

Goldberger's work in seeking out the cause of pellagra, of proving his theory in a series of fascinating experiments, and his pioneering efforts in pinpointing the exact dietary fault make up the bulk of this study. In this sense, it is part of the history of medicine and the history of nutrition. In a broader sense, however, it is a social history, for pellagra was irrevocably linked to the social and economic conditions of the early twentieth-century South. The frustration of those who saw pellagra as one of the most readily preventable diseases, but who watched the toll of its victims mount year after year because social and economic conditions were beyond the physicians' control, is part of this story. The agitation within the medical profession over accepting Goldberger's "strange" ideas, and the fury of the lay South over the stigma of poverty which his dietary theory implied, are other facets.

Research for this study was done primarily at the University of Georgia library, the National Archives in Washington, D.C., and the National Library of Medicine in Bethesda, Maryland. I am grateful to the staffs of these institutions for the help

they gave me, as well as to the staff of the Southern Historical
Collection at the University of North Carolina and the members
of the manuscripts division at the South Caroliniana Library
at Columbia, South Carolina, the Library of the Medical University of South Carolina at Charleston, and the Duke University
Library, all of whom were kind and helpful. Members of the
interlibrary loan division at Longwood College, Farmville, Virginia, were also unstinting in their efforts to secure material
for me. I am also grateful to Dr. Joseph Goldberger, Jr., of
El Reno, Oklahoma, who answered queries about his father's
work; to Dr. Ralph Chester Williams, now of Atlanta, Georgia,
who was for many years a member of the U.S. Public Health
Service staff and an associate of Goldberger, who granted me
a long interview; and to the late Dr. Rolla E. Dyer, director
of the National Institutes of Health from 1942 to 1950, who
told me about the pellagra investigations in South Carolina on
which he worked as a young man.

This book grew out of a doctoral dissertation in history written
at the University of Georgia in 1966. Many members of the
history faculty there offered constructive criticism. Professor
Horace Montgomery directed the study. Dedication of this book
to him expresses only in part my gratitude.

EWE

Farmville, Virginia
June 1971

The Butterfly Caste

1

A New Scourge
for the South

On a march day in 1902, a young, poor Georgia farmer went to Atlanta to seek advice and aid from a city physician. Spring had come, and, for the fifteenth consecutive year, the farmer showed signs of a strange and disabling warm weather sickness, which would probably cause his weight to drop to less than a hundred pounds, make his body burn as if on fire, and cause great blisters to appear on his arms and hands. It was a strange kind of "spring fever" which usually appeared before mid-February, gradually grew worse until May or June, and then began to abate. The patient was melancholy and depressed. His physician, Dr. H. F. Harris, was intrigued. Here, indeed, was an interesting case, and, if his diagnosis of pellagra were correct, it was the first case of the scourge that afflicted much of Europe to be reported in the United States. Unhappily for the young farmer, whose identity is not recorded, there was not much help that Harris could give him. He told him simply to move to a cooler climate and quit eating anything made from decomposed Indian corn.

This case history is interesting in that it recorded the fact that the patient had been brought up in unusual poverty and that he had always eaten bread made from Indian corn. Poverty and corn: these were the two factors that were to be cited often in the years to come when pellagra was widespread in the South and when doctors and laymen alike sought frantically for the cause and a cure.

A few weeks after Harris saw the farmer, he reported the case in some detail to a meeting of the Medical Association of Georgia.[1] His paper created almost no interest, and those members of the medical profession who cared to notice it at all marked it as merely a curiosity. Within five years, however, doctors throughout the South had cause to remember the Georgia farmer's strange illness. In neighboring Alabama, Dr. George H. Searcy diagnosed as acute pellagra the debilitating illness of eighty-eight inmates at the Mount Vernon Insane Hospital. There was an epidemic of it at this institution for Negroes in the summer of 1906, and the mortality rate was a shocking 64 percent. When this was reported to the Medical Association of Alabama in the spring of 1907, doctors in Alabama and throughout the South took notice.[2]

What was diagnosed as pellagra in 1906 was the same disease that had been appearing in a few patients at Mount Vernon every year since 1901. The disease usually had proved fatal; until 1906, however, it had not been recognized as a specific disease, but had simply been listed as a general debility. Searcy pinpointed the symptoms: rough, scaly skin in one or more locations and severe disturbances of the digestive tract and the nervous system. Significantly, he noted that the disease occurred among the poor and in institutions where the diet was at times limited, and he observed that it occurred much more frequently among women than men. The prognosis in acute cases was always unfavorable. Death could be expected in two to three weeks.

Like Harris, Searcy blamed the disease on the continuous eating of damaged corn. A sample of the cornmeal used at Mount Vernon was sent to Washington, D.C., for analysis where it was pronounced unfit for human consumption. The meal was made of moldy grain and contained rather large quantities of a variety of bacteria and fungi. Immediately, corn bread and grits were eliminated from the diet at Mount Vernon, and the patients were served wheat bread and potatoes instead. This new diet was much like that of the nurses at the institution, none of whom was sick. Within ten days, no new cases appeared among the inmates of Mount Vernon. But Searcy warned that much of the 1905 Western corn crop had been damaged by wet weather and that doctors should watch for the disease among their patients, especially among Negroes who often had little more to eat than corn bread and rarely had meat.[3]

Southern doctors, following Searcy's warning, looked for pellagra cases and found them. Dr. James Woods Babcock, superintendent of the State Hospital for the Insane at Columbia, South Carolina, soon reported nine suspected cases of the disease in that institution.[4] His paper on the subject, published in the *American Journal of Insanity*, aroused national concern. Pellagra was first noticed at the sprawling Georgia State Sanitarium in Milledgeville in 1908, when forty cases and twenty-three deaths were reported. Those afflicted ranged in age from six to seventy-five; nearly all who died were female. The superintendent of the hospital wrote in his annual report that the disease had probably occurred in the institution for years, but they had not known what to call it. Indeed, now that they had a name for it, they were no better off, for there was no specific "to cover its ravages."[5] That year tuberculosis was the leading cause of death at the Milledgeville hospital, and pellagra was second. A year later, pellagra was the number one killer there, causing seventy-three deaths, 16 percent of the hospital's total. Corn was suspect as its cause, and it was eliminated from the diets of anyone with symptoms of the disease. But the hospital had limited funds; it had to meet all its expenses on a budget of thirty-seven cents per patient per day, an amount too small to furnish much variety in diet. The superintendent noted they could not serve patients desserts and there was never enough milk.[6]

At the Louisiana Hospital for the Insane, the "peculiar and fatal" disease of 1907–1908 was pellagra; there were at least forty cases there during the spring and summer of 1909. By October of that year, the superintendent no longer could conscientiously serve corn bread and grits daily. These were eliminated from the diet, and, within four weeks, patients began to get well. Maniacal pellagrins became calm, and some appeared to be perfectly sane.[7]

There were also reports of pellagra in mental institutions in Virginia and Mississippi and, more surprising, in Illinois, where much corn was raised but relatively little was eaten. At the Peoria State Hospital in November 1909, there were 130 well-defined cases of the disease, which had caused forty-five deaths since mid-August. The superintendent, Dr. George A. Zeller, admitted that the discovery of pellagra there—the first cases found in the North—came as a shock; Illinois physicians had thought the state immune to it. The first case definitely diagnosed, plus the dozens of cases with similar symptoms, jogged memories of hospital officials. Zeller recalled that there had been an unusual amount of sunburn at the hospital in recent years, and one of the first signs of pellagra was reddened skin that looked so much like sunburn it was hard to tell them apart. They remembered patients who had died apparently after being scalded in the bathtub. These had been treated without success for second-degree burns, and the nurses who had attended them had been dismissed for negligence. Looking back, Zeller realized that the nurses who had stoutly denied any wrongdoing had been maligned. Pellagra, not hot water, had caused the ugly red ankles and the subsequent deaths.[8]

Not all the early reports of pellagra came from insane asylums. There were reports from orphanages, mill villages, cities, and rural areas. An orphanage in Decatur, Georgia, reported a dozen cases in 1911. Many children from mill villages in South Carolina were reported ill. The doctor who treated them for diarrhea and stomatitis—two early signs of pellagra—noted that nearly everybody in the village had the same complaint.[9]

Pellagra was at once both difficult and easy to diagnose. After the characteristic symmetrical lesions appeared on the hands and arms, on the tops of the feet and around the ankles, on the back of the neck or in a butterfly-shaped design across the nose, it was fairly easy to recognize pellagra. In its early stages, however, the reddening of the skin might be confused with sunburn or poison oak. It was not until the reddened skin began to crust and peel, revealing a smooth glossy skin underneath, that a certain diagnosis of pellagra could be made. "If you ever shake hands with one of these patients, you never forget the sensation," one South Carolina physician remarked. "The skin of the hand is dead, harsh, and rough." Without skin symptoms, however, a pellagra case was like an unsigned letter. The skin symptom was the signature identifying the disease. Some pellagra victims showed no skin symptoms. They had only a disturbance of the digestive tract or such vague symptoms as a general feeling of malaise, listlessness, weak knees, pain in the back and neck, or an uncertainty of motion much like that of a beginner on roller skates. Very often there was a severe burning sensation in the stomach and extremities, especially the feet. The mouth became extremely sore and the tongue glossy and inflamed. The victim might suffer from either diarrhea or constipation, although diarrhea was more common. Usually the rather vague symptoms of distress began shortly after Christmas, with more definite signs of the disease appearing in the spring. Erythema—the reddening of both hands, both feet, or a symmetrical design on the back of the neck or the face—might occur as early as March or April, or as late as June. Some cases were chronic, occurring about the same time year after year and then disappearing in the late summer and fall. Others were acute, developed rapidly, and ended fatally within a few weeks.[10]

The mind could be severely affected. Patients were often melancholy or suffered from delusions of persecution. They seldom laughed, were frequently confused, could not tell the truth, and had hallucinations. Illusions of pregnancy were fairly common among insane women pellagrins. Some had destructive tendencies; they might pull out their eyebrows or try to set their houses on fire. Others feared for their safety, imagining that the neighbors planned to assassinate them.

One of the more serious aspects of the insane pellagra victim's behavior was his penchant for suicide. Among women in particular, water held an especially fatal attraction as the suicidal method. Nurses in asylums had to watch carefully to keep women patients from drowning themselves in the bathtub. Patients were known to weight their clothing down with stones and jump into a well or pond. Men showed greater variety in suicidal methods. At least one threw himself under a train; another drank carbolic acid; and a third beat his head against a wall. So frequently was pellagra associated with suicide that in 1915, when the number of cases of pellagra reached its highest peak in Mississippi, the 120 percent increase in the number of suicides in the state that year was attributed to the sharp jump in the incidence of pellagra.[11]

Contributing to the terror of pellagra was a belief by some physicians that the disease, horrible enough in itself, was rendered the more awful because it very likely was hereditary. Not many believed it was communicable, but the belief that it could be passed from one generation to the next was common. One Georgia doctor commented that pellagra "carries death and despair in its very name." He was convinced that the poisoning effects of the disease were not spent just on the individual subject, but were transferred to the next generation, and he was afraid that if the infection became firmly rooted it would "manifest its baneful influence forever upon the human family."[12] Pellagra rapidly became known as the disease of the four D's: diarrhea, dermatitis, dementia, and death.

At first, it seemed that pellagra had appeared from nowhere to bring fear and desolation to the South. After the initial surprise, however, there were many doctors, who, like the superintendent at the Peoria State Hospital, had their memories jogged. They remembered earlier cases, and a search of the records turned up evidence that pellagra had probably existed in the United States for years. Dr. Babcock at the Hospital for the Insane in Columbia took the most active interest in this historical search. He found in the files of his institution the case history of a man admitted in 1834 who showed every sign of pellagra. A careful search of the literature showed isolated cases reported in New York and Massachusetts in 1864 and others in Brooklyn in 1882 and 1902. In 1916, Dr. W. J. Kerr, the surgeon who had been in charge of Andersonville Prison during the Civil War, even said that it was probably pellagra, not typhoid, that caused the hundreds of deaths there in the summer of 1864.[13]

One of the reasons why American physicians had failed to diagnose pellagra before 1907–1908 was that the disease simply had not been recognized. A well-known medical text, Austin Flint's *A Treatise on the Principles and Practices of Medicine* (1866–1894), did not mention it at all. John Herr Musser's *A Practical Treatise on Medical Diagnosis* (1894–1913), ignored it until the fifth edition (1904), when it was given one paragraph under "grain poisonings." The first seven editions of Sir William Osler's *The Principles and Practice of Medicine* (1892–1909), gave it but scant notice, saying that it had not been observed in the United States. Illnesses that Southern physicians had once inexactly called foot-and-mouth disease, and tubercular enteritis, solar dermatitis, or black gloves disease were relabeled pellagra.[14]

Although it was a stranger in America, pellagra had long been known in Europe. Don Gaspar Casál, a physician in the Spanish court, first described it in 1735. Among the peasants of Asturias he noted a peculiar kind of leprosy known as *mal de la rosa*. "Since I never saw a more disgusting indigenous disease," he wrote, "I thought I should explain its characteristics."[15] There followed the classic description of the disease with its extreme weakness, sensations of burning, crusts on the skin, and melancholia. Casál's associate at court, the French physician François Thiéry, actually published the first account of the disease. His paper, stating that *mal de la rosa* resisted all remedies, appeared in a French journal in 1755. Casál's account was published posthumously in 1762. Less than ten years later, the disease was noted in Italy, and an Italian physician, Francesco Frapolli, published a careful account and gave the disease the name pellagra.[16]

Foreign travelers in Italy and Spain also commented on pellagra, occasionally suggesting a possible cause or a cure. An English clergyman traveling in Spain in 1786 wrote that *mal de la rosa* could be cured by nitre and gentle cathartics but, if neglected, it terminated in "scrophula, marasma, melancholia, and madness." The German poet Goethe wrote that same year from Italy that he was much displeased by the pale brownish complexion of the women there. He attributed their sickly condition to the frequent consumption of Indian corn and buckwheat, which they ground and made into a pap with water. They did not eat meat, he noted: "This necessarily glues up and stops the alimentary channels, especially with the women and children, and their cachetic complexion is an indication of the malady."[17]

Casál had wondered if the cause of the disease were to be sought in the heavens, the condition of the atmosphere, or in the constitution or diet of the patients. He soon ruled out a faulty diet, although he noted that maize was the chief article of diet of pellagrins and that they rarely ate meat. Later students of the disease, however, decided that diet was the most important factor and that maize was the leading offender. The first definite theory connecting corn with pellagra was formulated in 1810 when the Italian Dr. Giovanni Battista Marzari suggested that pellagra was due to a lack of certain nutritive elements in corn. Not even Marzari realized how far ahead of his time he was. Two schools of thought arose: the Zeists

(from *zea mays,* the botanical name of maize) who supported
Marzari, and the anti-Zeists who discredited his theory. Within
a few years, the Zeists complicated matters with a split among
themselves. The accusing finger then was pointed not at good
sound corn which lacked some mysterious nutritive element, but
at spoiled corn, which might be guilty because of the variety
of fungi and bacteria it contained.

Lodovico Balardini, another Italian physician, discovered cop-
per-green moulds growing on spoiled corn in 1844. He believed
these moulds created a toxic substance that, if taken into the
body long enough, would produce pellagra. His accusations
against spoiled corn were seconded with enthusiasm a few years
later by Cesare Lombroso of Turin, a squat, bespectacled doctor
as much interested in criminology as medicine, who became
the leading advocate of the spoiled corn theory. He spent the
next twenty-five years studying the various moulds and bacteria
that grew on damp corn, trying without success to pinpoint
a single factor that caused the disease. The common blue mould,
penicillium glaucum, was most often found on spoiled corn,
and so was most often accused. Lombroso made an alcoholic
extract from damaged maize, which he called *Pellagrazine.* When
injected into men or animals, it produced symptoms of the disease. Lombroso was also the first to suggest that arsenic be used
in treating pellagra. Like his spoiled corn idea, the arsenic treatment was widely and enthusiastically adopted.[18]

By the early twentieth century still another Italian, Guido
Tizzoni, announced triumphantly that he had at last isolated
the true cause of pellagra. He obtained pure cultures of a specific
bacillus from the blood and fecal matter of pellagrins and injected it into guinea pigs that promptly died. "It would seem
to be settled that pellagra is a bacterial disease," he wrote.
Strangely, the new organism, named *streptobacillus pellagrae,*
did not cause illness in guinea pigs that had eaten no corn.
Sound corn was thus condemned anew as a predisposing influence in pellagra. *Streptobacillus pellagrae* could not even be

destroyed by cooking. It readily withstood temperatures of 194 degrees Fahrenheit for an hour without injury.[19]

In the summer of 1908, the new scourge of the South was definitely identified as the same disease as the long-recognized Italian pellagra. Babcock, superintendent of the South Carolina Hospital for the Insane, took a recreational tour of Europe that year with his long-time friend, South Carolina's Senator Benjamin R. "Pitchfork Ben" Tillman. In Italy, they visited several hospitals for pellagrins, where Babcock became convinced that the two diseases on opposite sides of the Atlantic were the same. The Senator, no authority on medicine, was impressed by the poverty of the people and what he called their "horrible lack of pride." He was also sufficiently impressed with the danger that pellagra posed in the United States to request the American vice-consul in Milan to prepare a complete report on pellagra in Italy and what the government was doing to control it.[20]

Back in Columbia, the South Carolina Board of Health instigated a thorough investigation of pellagra. In October, Babcock suggested that there were enough pellagra cases at the State Hospital to furnish material for a meaningful study. The conference was arranged, and late that month, seventy-two physicians, all but eight of them from South Carolina, met in the South Carolina Hospital for the Insane to share what information they had on the mysterious disease.[21] Among the speakers were Senator Tillman and a representative from the United States Public Health Service, Dr. Claude H. Lavinder, who was to assume an important role in the pellagra investigations in the months to come.

Public reaction throughout the country to reports of the increasing number of pellagra cases was mixed. Some physicians treated it as a joke. Most doctors had never encountered pellagra in their practice, and many viewed it as some exotic scourge like sleeping sickness. There were others, however, who were concerned. Searcy, who had first spotted the disease at Mount Vernon Insane Hospital, thought there was great probability the disease would spread. Believing it to be based solely on corn bread and poverty, Searcy reasoned that, as the population increased, there would be a corresponding rise in both poverty and the consumption of corn bread. Pellagra would naturally follow. A North Carolina physician called it an "utterly hopeless disease." Babcock said it posed the greatest sanitary problem in modern times, and a Texas doctor estimated that there were 2 million cases in the United States.[22]

The stories about pellagra in the public press were not calculated to soothe the troubled. In November 1909, *McClure's* magazine published a rather sensational article, "A Medical Mystery," which recounted the horrors of the disease, announced that it was hereditary, affecting even the third and fourth generations, and warned the well-to-do that they were not immune. In America, the writer pointed out, pellagra attacked rich and poor alike. Another national journal, *Good Health,* compared pellagra to bubonic plague; the plague was pictured as less fearsome. Some Southerners, ever sensitive to attacks on the culture of the South, believed the whole pellagra question was agitated merely to inflict further injury on a besieged land, but there were others equally convinced that another loathsome and fatal malady had indeed taken hold.[23]

Pellagra was the second serious disease peculiar to the South to be discovered within a period of a few years. Almost simultaneously, the widespread prevalence of hookworm in the region had brought national attention and outside help as well. More than 2 million cases of hookworm, or the "lazy man's disease" as it was dubbed by the Northern press, were scattered across the South. In 1909, John D. Rockefeller made a million-dollar gift to Southern states to be used over a period of five years to eradicate the disease. Though peculiarly associated with the geography and climate of the South, hookworm was also related to the sanitary habits of Southern life, and its eradication required not only medical treatment but a massive educational campaign as well. Easy enough to diagnose, and curable with a few cents worth of thymol, hookworm would keep reappearing unless several million people could be convinced to improve their sanitary habits. To bring about such a change, as *The State* of Columbia, S.C., observed, was an "arduous task, and will require the cooperation of boards of health, physicians, county commissioners, and school teachers."[24]

Not all Southerners were ready to offer instant cooperation with the Rockefeller Sanitary Commission. As a rule, the medical profession backed the commission's efforts fully, but there was much doubt at the beginning of the campaign as to how the public would react. Since hookworms entered the body through the feet, there were rumors that the commission had started the hookworm scare so that the Southern population would wear shoes; the commission would then get rich selling shoes. Some considered it an insult to suggest that Southern people had worms. A repulsive idea, this seemed to strike at Southern pride. Methodist Bishop Warren A. Candler was incensed that Rockefeller had advertised the South as a center of that "horrid hookworm."

Despite this evidence of prejudice, however, the campaign made fairly good progress. The massive effort against hookworm coincided exactly with the early efforts to combat pellagra, but the hookworm campaign was much more successful. Hookworm disease was much simpler to diagnose; its cause was something that could be seen under a microscope; a cure was not only known, it was cheap. The average cost of treating each patient was fifty-six cents. The public, after a little educational priming, embraced the antihookworm campaign heartily. Atlanta conducted an intensive bond campaign in 1910 to raise $3 million for sanitary improvements. Public schools were used to distribute information; the press was very effective. And the Southern public was so fascinated that some people walked fifteen or twenty miles to a hookworm dispensary station. They enjoyed looking at slides and charts, and would wait in line for two hours to look at a hookworm larvae and a mature worm under the microscope. More important, they did change their sanitary habits. When the commission or the local health departments provided guidance on the building of new sanitary privies, Southerners built them and were proud of their efforts. Officials of the sanitary commission believed the most important element in the success of the eradication campaign was the overwhelming support of the Southern people.[25]

The campaign against pellagra was to be a beneficiary of the antihookworm campaign. As a result of the emphasis on eradicating hookworm, county health departments were established throughout the South. These local health agencies were almost nonexistent in 1910, but by 1917, they were flourishing. Appropriations for statewide health work were also increased as a result of the interest in hookworm. In 1910, the budget for the eleven Southern states included under the Rockefeller program was $216,195. In 1918, it was $1,316,111, an increase of 454 percent in less than ten years.[26] Through these state and local agencies, much of the fight against pellagra was to be waged.

Pellagra, wrapped in mystery as it was, was a more frightening disease than hookworm, and doctors and laymen alike maintained a hopeful stance only with difficulty. In fact, the only cheerful attitude toward the outbreak of pellagra in the United States was taken by an Englishman, Dr. F. M. Sandwith of the Society of Tropical Medicine and Hygiene. The news that pellagra had invaded the American South came as no surprise. He had discovered pellagra among maize-eating peasants in Egypt, Italy, and South Africa. Knowing of the consumption of maize in the Southern United States, he suspected pellagra existed there, too. With his suspicions finally confirmed, he wrote that the world waited in the "confident hope" that the long unsolved pellagra problems would be successfully mastered in the United States. The chief threat he saw to eventual success was that "enterprising" people in the South would diagnose everything as "doubtful pellagra." If that happened, he warned, the whole pellagra question would fall into disrepute. Sandwith's confidence in American ability was well founded. Pellagra was to be stripped of its secrets in America, largely through the efforts of the United States Public Health Service.[27]

Soon after pellagra was first reported at the Mount Vernon Insane Hospital, the Public Health Service began its antipellagra campaign; it got off to a slow start. A staff member from the Marine Hospital at Mobile, Alabama, was directed merely to investigate the situation at Mount Vernon and prepare a brief report without incurring expense. A year later little additional action had been taken, but, at the urging of Searcy who wrote both his congressman and the Surgeon General that pellagra posed a more serious problem in the South than hookworm, malaria, or tuberculosis, the PHS began to take a more active interest. The Public Health Services' C. H. Lavinder, in a tour of the South, encountered many cases and noted the need for an educational campaign. "Knowledge of the disease is certainly possessed by but few American physicians," he wrote Surgeon General Walter Wyman, "and to most it is hardly a name." In Lavinder's opinion, the PHS should view the disease from the public health standpoint. It was a large question which would require, among other things, an investigation of the corn crop and its methods of culture in the United States. The prospects for good results from such a study were doubtful at best, Lavinder wrote, but it was one that must be undertaken. The Surgeon General was stirred to action. Warning that pellagra threatened to become a scourge in the South, he appointed a seven-man commission to investigate the disease in all its facets.[28]

The Public Health Service began serious work at the South Carolina Hospital for the Insane in May 1909, where two small rooms had been set aside for a laboratory. The rooms had neither water nor gas, but Lavinder, who was in charge of the work there, was satisfied that in time these laboratory essentials would be provided. Meanwhile, he began work as best he could. Certainly, there was no shortage of material with which to work. There were a number of cases of pellagra in the hospital itself and many more in the surrounding city and county. Lavinder followed experimental lines pursued by the Italian investigators: he injected rabbits, rats, chickens, and guinea pigs with the blood, spinal fluid, and spleen pulp of pellagrins, hoping to induce the disease. He got only negative results.

As Lavinder worked, he became more convinced that pellagra constituted a grave threat to the South. Because diagnosis was difficult, he suspected that there were many more cases than had been reported. "The sick are pitiful and too often loathsome objects," he wrote. Treatment was ineffective, especially in asylum cases. The afflicted lay for days or even weeks in bed with an extensive purulent condition of the skin on the hands, feet, or neck, frequent diarrhea, deep mental depression, bed sores, and marked emaciation.[29]

During the summer Lavinder spent at the hospital, he checked the blood of pellagrins and found them anemic. He tried experimental therapy with salts of mercury and arsenic and with serum from the blood of recovered pellagrins. He examined specimens, conducted autopsies, and made hurried trips to Illinois and Tennessee where there were pellagra outbreaks. His was a one-man operation. Lavinder had no expert assistance and no clerical help.

The next spring, a second member of the Pellagra Commission was sent to Columbia in Lavinder's place. Dr. John D. Long had little patience with Southern folkways, which often delayed research. The work was an "uphill kind," Long observed, because the people were so slow and easygoing. It took two days to get a stool to the laboratory for examination and three days to a week for a blood count. He complained, too, that except for Babcock and one other doctor in Columbia, there were no local doctors who took any interest in pellagra or in anything else. "I do not know whether it is the heat or hookworm, or whether they were born that way," he wrote.[30]

In spite of these difficulties, however, Long made some

progress. He found that pellagrins had marked indigestion, that most were infected with roundworms, hookworms, whipworms, or amoebas and that many showed joint changes much like those caused by arthritis. After inspecting an outbreak of beriberi among convicts at Charleston, one of whom also had symptoms of pellagra, he suggested that pellagra and beriberi were related. Long suspected that poor sanitary conditions were a factor in causing the disease. He investigated an outbreak of pellagra at Columbus, Georgia, and reported that sanitary conditions there were poor. His favorite treatment for pellagrins was rest in bed, a diet of milk, well-toasted bread, and soft-cooked rice, followed by five grains of pancreatin after meals to aid digestion. Prevention of the disease seemed to resolve itself into one thing, he wrote the Surgeon General: sanitation. If the danger of parasitic infection could be removed and the people taught to eat a more diverse diet not so rich in protein, pellagra would disappear.[31]

The most dramatic event in the early years of the antipellagra campaign was the first National Conference on Pellagra held in Columbia, November 3–4, 1909. Headquarters for this conference, like the smaller one a year earlier, was the State Hospital for the Insane. Babcock was again the organizer, and the conference was a success. There were approximately two hundred physicians present for the opening sessions of the two-day meeting, and, before it was finished, a total of 394 had registered. They came from nearly every state and from many countries. Columbia was crowded with doctors.

When the conference was planned, Babcock thought it would be of interest only in South Carolina, so, to benefit local physicians, the date was set for the same week as the state fair. But the word spread. Hotel accommodations in Columbia, limited at best, were severely overtaxed, and many delegates were housed on the grounds of the state hospital. The large attendance boosted hopes that good results might come from the conference, and added to the lustre which it was believed the conference gave to Columbia's name. Sessions were extensively covered, not only by the local press, but by reporters from out of the state as well. *The* (Columbia) *State* commented that, despite the fact there was little local interest in the convention, it was the biggest story for the entire country that had originated in Columbia in years and that it was watched throughout America. The meeting was dubbed a "big thing in health history"; it was attended by "big men." The local press did its part to stimulate interest in pellagra. *The State,* for example, ran pictures of the speakers, included complete texts of the speeches, and at least once gave the conference a whole-page spread.

Papers read at the conference covered every known aspect of the pellagra question, and, according to one reporter, were "verbose and difficult to be understood." Certainly, there was no consensus on the cause or cure of pellagra but no one at the conference anticipated immediate results. As one Virginia physician commented, "it would be absurd to expect that America in a year could crack the nut that had been a practical impossibility in Europe for a hundred years."[32]

The conference did organize the National Association for the Study of Pellagra and named Babcock, who had already acquired a reputation as an innovator in the care of the insane, as its first president. Fifteen years earlier, Babcock had been the first to urge isolation and modern care for tuberculosis patients in these institutions. The Columbia conference recognized him officially as the "father of the movement for the study and control of pellagra in America."[33]

Babcock was one of South Carolina's most distinguished physicians. A graduate of Harvard College and Harvard Medical School, he had been superintendent of the State Hospital for the Insane since 1891. He had distinguished himself as a psychiatrist—then called alienist—and, although he operated the state hospital on a tiny budget, was able to practice advanced therapy in mental illness, including the still new methods of Sigmund Freud. After discovering the existence of pellagra in the hospital in 1907, he spent much of his time working on the disease. A few months before the Columbia conference, the South Carolina Medical Association unanimously adopted a resolution in appreciation of his discovery of the disease in the state. Because of his interest in pellagra, physicians from a wide area consulted him, and pellagrins came in large numbers asking for help. Babcock set aside every Sunday for consultations on pellagra, for which he never charged a fee. Instead, although his salary was small, he spent some $2,000 of his own money on the study of pellagra during the half-dozen years after he discovered the disease in the hospital. It was Babcock's work with pellagra that had prompted Senator Tillman's concern. The Senator had one of Babcock's more popular papers on the subject, "The Prevalence of Pellagra in the United States," printed as a public document in 1911.[34]

While the conference did not formally pinpoint the cause of pellagra, it very strongly implicated corn, especially spoiled corn. Though there was only circumstantial evidence against it, corn seemed always to be present wherever there was pellagra. Lavinder pointed out that pellagra closely followed the introduction of maize culture into Spain, France, Italy, and other countries of southern Europe. Only where maize was extensively grown was pellagra an endemic disease.[35]

The reaction to the indictment of corn was immediate. Corn was the principal crop of the country and big money was involved; marketing of the crop both at home and abroad was endangered. To cite corn as the cause of pellagra could be a stinging blow to the nation's purse. There was so much correspondence with the United States Department of Agriculture about pellagra that the department launched an investigation on the economic phases of the question. There were studies on the growing, curing, transporting, milling, and marketing of corn and corn products and the conditions which caused spoiling.[36] Southern states launched their own investigations on corn to determine if the "death dealing qualities" charged against it were developed in the home-raised goods or in the corn brought in from other states. The Commissioner of Agriculture of South Carolina was so concerned over the corn–pellagra issue that he said that a million dollars spent against pellagra would be more valuable than Rockefeller's princely gift against hookworm. South Carolina alone, he pointed out, grew 30 million bushels of the grain, yet still spent $6 million outside the state for corn, not including expenditures for grits, meal, corn-flakes, cornstarch, yeast, and corn whiskey. The Southern market for Western corn was certainly important enough for Western growers to wish to protect it. The *Chicago Post* commented that if Southern millers or their customers ever "get it into their heads that Illinois corn is the cause of pellagra, we shall feel the economic effect of it in this state, world wide though our markets be."[37]

Talk of the elimination of grits and corn bread from the diet had many repercussions. It even gave temperance leaders a new stage for their continuing war on alcohol. Rumors were rife that corn liquor and beer were made from corn that was otherwise unfit for use, and it was a well-known fact that some heavy drinkers had pellagra. *Good Health* magazine even singled out beer as the most constant source of the disease. It charged that corn not good enough to be ground into grits or meal was made into beer, and thus beer drinkers ran a far greater risk of contracting pellagra than those who used corn in the ordinary way. "If the discovery of pellagra has the effect to materially lessen the consumption of beer," the *Good Health* editor wrote, "it may be the means of accomplishing great good in the battle against intemperance."[38]

Large segments of the public accepted as fact that musty corn caused pellagra, and there were widespread demands that the South grow enough corn to meet its own needs. If corn were grown and milled at home and carefully inspected, there would be no danger of musty meal finding its way to the market. It was argued that home-grown corn not only would protect

Experts from the United States Department of Agriculture (USDA), investigating the relationship between corn and pellagra, suggested that a succession of cold, wet falls may have been responsible for the outbreak of the disease. Indian summer weather was deemed essential for the proper maturing of corn, and, for almost a decade, the Indian summers had been short. These experts also suggested that corn culture had been pushed north rapidly where the chances of unsuitable weather for the ripening of corn were thus increased. They added that it was even possible that the northern limit for safe corn culture had been exceeded. Sound corn might also be spoiled by poor methods of shipment. Put in closed cars with no ventilation, the corn gave off heat and fungi developed. If the corn were shipped to the Northeast, they reasoned, the cooler weather checked the growth of the fungi; if it were shipped to the South where the weather was warm, fungus growth was encouraged.[40]

Whatever the reasons for spoiled corn, the outcry against it was shrill. A Maryland physician stated flatly that two-thirds of the cases of pellagra could be attributed to the corn harvester; one from Virginia called pellagra the "corn curse," a disease caused by a demon which lurks in a green fungus. The fungus might attack the corn at any time: in the field, in the crib, at the mill, before or after grinding, and even after cooking, if left for any length of time. He therefore advised that no cold corn bread should ever be used for food and that breakfast cereal made from corn should be carefully examined. To insure that bad corn be kept off the market, he recommended that millers grinding musty corn and storekeepers selling musty meal be fined and imprisoned.[41]

In some areas, there was insistent demand for inspection laws, which would keep damaged corn off the market. In Italy, where pellagra once had been prevalent, stringent inspection laws had been passed to prevent the marketing of spoiled corn, and special desiccating plants had been established for the artificial drying of the grain.[42] The incidence of the disease had dropped rather dramatically in Italy, and Americans saw here an object lesson. Inspection of grain was thought to be desirable not only because it might prevent pellagra but also because there was no good reason to consume spoiled corn. The USDA set up specifications for high-grade corn: not more than 12 percent moisture nor more than 30 percent acidity. The agricultural experts made no claim that spoiled corn caused pellagra. They did claim that dealers in moist corn had overreached themselves, causing the price of American corn on the world's market to tumble and practically closing some of these markets to one of the nation's most important crops.[43]

There were some Southerners who would have liked to have closed their state markets to Western corn. In 1911 the secretary of the Georgia State Board of Health recommended that the state prohibit the importation of all Western corn into Georgia. He claimed there were 50,000 cases of pellagra in the South. The next year the Georgia Health Board circulated a bulletin solemnly warning the people of the state against eating Western corn "so long as the pernicious practice continues of cultivating a weakened and vitiated plant, combined with a method of harvesting which is nothing less than criminal." Health officials called again for legislation to stop the murder of Georgia citizens and the slaughter of the state's horses by sale of corn unfit for consumption. A professor at the state College of Agriculture in Athens said that Western corn cut green was in every particular bad.[44]

North Carolinians also demanded corn inspection laws so that they might eat corn bread without fear, and Texans asked for congressional action to control the sale of musty corn. The outcry against musty corn was greatest in South Carolina and there, largely because of the efforts of an energetic Commissioner of Agriculture, E. J. Watson, an inspection law was passed and enforced.[45] It was the only state to have such control over the corn market. The interest in pellagra in South Carolina was intense. The report of the Board of Health of South Carolina said in 1910 that "no disease in the history of the State had ever aroused so much interest among both the members of the medical profession and the laity alike as has that of pellagra. That the disease is a serious one, there is no doubt."[46]

Not everyone blamed the outbreak of pellagra on new harvesting methods. Some people believed that Italian immigrants brought into the South to cut timber had brought pellagra with them. Pellagra and the "stave-getters itch" the Italians suffered from were the same disease, they said. The outcry against Italians was sharp enough to force United States immigration officers in Italy to refuse Italian pellagrins entry to the United States for health reasons. Pellagra was also blamed on spring heat and sunshine, on the "delicacy" of women's nervous systems, and even on the emancipation of the slaves. Negroes, a Georgia physician insisted, had many more diseases, including pellagra, since emancipation, than they had before. He considered the increased insanity among Negroes alarming.[47]

A pellagra germ was actively sought. This was the era when bacteriologists throughout the world had made such dramatic progress in discovering causes of diseases that scientists were often blinded to other avenues of thought. Since 1876, when the German Robert Koch proved that a bacillus caused anthrax, the mystery had been stripped from one infectious disease after another. Koch himself discovered the bacteria causing tuberculosis in 1882, and, within the next quarter-century, the pathogenic bacteria of cholera, diphtheria, typhoid, tetanus, bubonic plague, and syphilis had all been unmasked. Tropical dysentery could be blamed with certainty on an amoeba, and cattle contracted "Texas fever" when bitten by an infected tick. Dramatic experiments in the late 1890s by a British physician, Ronald Ross, in the Indian medical service, and by the Italian Battista Grazzi, proved that the anopheles mosquito carried the malaria parasite. Coming out of the Spanish-American war was the dramatic story of how a group of Johns Hopkins men, led by Walter Reed, had found the origin of yellow fever epidemics in the bite of another mosquito, the *stegomyia fasciata*. It was thus natural that the search for the cause of pellagra should take a similar course.

At the height of the pellagra scare in the United States, Dr. Louis Sambon of the London School of Tropical Medicine, advanced the theory that pellagra was a waterborne disease, disseminated by an insect, probably the simulium or buffalo gnat.[48] This was good news to the boosters of American agriculture. An article in *The American Agriculturist* gave an account of Sambon's theory under the heading, "Pellagra, Insect-Borne?" and commented with satisfaction that this seemed to refute the idea that pellagra might be caused by musty corn.[49] There were serious objections to the simulium theory in America, however. The bite of the fly was poisonous rather than infectious; the simulium never moved far from its home on rapidly moving streams, while pellagra victims often did not live near such streams; and the simulium was more numerous in cold countries than in warm.

If the mosquito were the carrier, there would be no such incongruities to explain away. Attacks of the disease coincided with the appearance of mosquitoes from the early spring to the fall; there were more mosquitoes—and more pellagra cases—in rural areas than in the cities; women were victims more often than men because, as stay-at-homes, they presumably (according to the reasoning) had more contact with the insects. Pellagra patients, were, therefore, advised to be well screened against mosquitoes, not to protect themselves from bites, but rather to deny the mosquitoes access to the pallagrous parasites believed to be circulating in their own blood.[50]

Despite high hopes, the search for a pellagra-producing germ was no more productive than the search for a toxin in corn. When one was not located in the bloodstream, it was proposed that perhaps the organisms were located in the brain or spinal cord. With the intensive hookworm eradication campaign underway in the South, it was not surprising that some doctors should advance the theory that pellagra, like hookworm, was caused by an intestinal parasite. The leading exponent of this theory was Dr. John L. Jelks of Memphis who found amoebas in most of his pellagra patients and was convinced that these amoebas carried with them bacteria or toxins, which found their way into the blood or lymph channels. He located what he believed to be the offending amoeba. People got pellagra, he said, by drinking polluted water or by eating infected vegetables.[51]

Even birds, especially blackbirds, were blamed as carriers of pellagra. It was argued that the blackbirds, while wintering in South America, picked up a pellagra-producing protozoan from horses which had a disease called *trypanosoma equinum,* an affliction not unlike pellagra in man. Flying north in the spring, the blackbirds stopped in the Southern United States, where the deadly *trypanosoma* in their bloodstreams were transmitted from bird to man by the bites of mosquitoes or flies or by the ingestion of cysts deposited by insects on plants. No *trypanosoma* had been found in the blood of human pellagrins, but, as the propounder of the blackbird theory told the American Medical Association in 1912, some were sure to be located soon.[52]

There was yet another school of thought on the etiology of pellagra. Two items in the Southern diet almost as popular as cornmeal, sugarcane products and cottonseed oil, were blamed. The charge against cane sugar was weightier because it was advanced by a physician of wide reputation, Dr. William Edgar Deeks of the Isthmian Canal Commission. Deeks had achieved fame for formulas for feeding babies and for success in treating nutritional diseases of the tropics. He said that corn or any starchy food eaten in connection with cane sugar in warm climates could lead to pellagra. Lessened metabolic activity in warm climates initiated the autointoxication, which was responsible for the disease. If his theory were correct, increased consumption of sugar in the South would cause a corresponding increase in pellagra. Deek's indictment of cane sugar met much opposition when it was first expressed in 1912, but it picked up a few followers in the years to come.[53]

An Atlanta physician, Dr. George C. Mizell, thought consumption of cottonseed oil caused pellagra. Although this idea received little or no support from the medical profession, there was much ado about it. The sizable cottonseed oil industry was disturbed; olive oil importers tried to use the furor as an entering wedge to boost their own product; and medical men like Lavinder, who had serious studies on pellagra underway, were annoyed at this new distraction.[54]

Mizell's theory was a novel one based on the widespread substitution of cottonseed oil shortening for lard in the South. According to Mizell, linolein, the characteristic fat of cottonseed oil, was unstable and unfit to perform the functions of normal animal fatty tissue. If it remained in the body for any length of time, it could cause pellagra. The physiological law governing the deposit of fats, he said, caused the face and hands to be affected more often than other parts of the body. Fats containing linolein were more liquid and thus were transported to the extremities. Oils similar to cottonseed oil which might have caused pellagra in the past, according to Mizell, were those of pumpkin seed, corn, kapok, sesame or benneseed, Brazil nuts, poppy seed, sunflowers, and walnuts.[55]

Quite naturally, the cottonseed oil industry rushed to the defense of its product. The processing of cottonseed oil involved the use of caustic soda, high temperatures, and several filtering processes. To company officials, it did not seem possible that a disease germ could endure this treatment. The industry strongly suspected that the whole cottonseed oil–pellagra theory was a plot planned by opposing commercial interests. In some areas circulars were even distributed citing cottonseed oil as the definite cause of the disease.[56]

The Public Health Service in time refuted the charges against cottonseed oil. Lavinder was particularly incensed about the attack on another wholesome article of food. "My candid opinion of [Mizell's theory] . . . can hardly be expressed with patience," he wrote the Surgeon General. According to Lavinder, it was ambiguous, full of errors, and contributed to the already potent wave of pellagraphobia.[57]

Alcoholism was commonly associated with pellagra as was a poor diet, but little significance was attached to the latter. One South Carolina physician, who discovered the disease among the Negroes cultivating the rice fields, observed that they needed "meat, red meat, and a variety of vegetables," but he was more concerned with the fact that they had eaten damp grits recovered from a flatboat which had sunk.[58] In spite of an occasional appearance of pellagra among the well-to-do, it was nearly always associated with poverty, breaking out among the poorly clothed, badly housed, and miserably fed.

In the early search for the cause of pellagra, there was no organized, concerted effort, a factor which contributed to the diversity of results. The Southern Medical Association cheered on the contestants in this scientific race. It held out as reward for the winner—the discoverer of pellagra's specific origin—the association's research medal. It fervently hoped that a Southerner, one of the association's own members, would win the prize.[59]

As pellagra spread rapidly across the South, there was a rising sense of panic. Records showed there were 15,870 cases in eight states of the South from 1907 through 1911, with a death rate of 39.1 percent. While fewer than 1,000 cases were reported in 1907, there were 7,000 or more in 1911.[60] It was the leading cause of death in the South's hospitals for the insane. A statewide conference was convened in Kentucky in 1911 to discuss the gravity of the problem there, and that same year so many cases appeared in Tennessee that the state appointed a Pellagra Commission to investigate. The *Journal of the American Medical Association* reported pellagra in more than thirty-two states and expressed concern that pellagra might become epidemic. Newspapers reported the mortality rate running as high as 80 percent, called the rapid spread of the disease alarming, and described it as a loathsome malady which brought death in its most horrible form: "Victims pass away in great agony, the pain being like pouring boiling water on wounds already scalded." Pellagra is too soothing a name for the disease, *The Greensboro* (North Carolina) *News* noted: "were we to speak of it as leprosy, the whole country would be crying out in wild alarm."[61]

The Public Health Service pleaded in vain for some sort of mental balance as hysterical cries went out to abandon the use of all corn, sound or unsound, and as victims of the disease were shunned as lepers, and isolated or quarantined. There was even some panic in the North when, as sporadic cases of pellagra appeared, newspapers called it "Italian leprosy," warned against consumption of corn (including corn whiskey), and advised readers that the malady might also be caused by using "other grains or other plant stuffs."[62]

Such vague warnings about what not to eat were the stuff of which pellagraphobia was made. Pellagra seemed too subtle a foe to be dealt with rationally, and public reaction to it was in some ways reminiscent of panic in a smallpox epidemic when so many flee that barely enough well people are left behind to care for the sick. In the case of pellagra, entire communities were not abandoned in a wild hegira, but victims were sometimes left as much alone as if this had been the case. So great was the horror of the disease that a diagnosis of pellagra was synonymous with a sentence of ostracism. A severe case of eczema was enough to start a stampede in a community, and pellagrins sometimes covered their hands with gloves or salve, hoping to conceal their condition.[63]

Many hospitals refused admission to pellagra patients. One in Atlanta did so on the grounds that it was an incurable disease. At another hospital in the same city, student nurses went on strike when they were required to nurse pellagrins. Physicians and nurses at Johns Hopkins Hospital in Baltimore were forbidden even to discuss pellagra cases which might be there. Fear of the disease spread to schools and hotels, too. One woman with an extremely mild case was staying at a family-type hotel in Atlanta while being treated by her physician. When word of her illness became known among the other guests, there was a unanimous demand to the hotel manager: the lady must go or everyone else would move out. In Centerville, Maryland, after two children in one family died of pellagra, the school-teacher attempted to bar other children in the family from school.[64]

Appearance of pellagra at Baptist Orphanage in Nashville, Tennessee, so alarmed the public that it was feared violence would erupt if the children were not moved from the hospital where they were being treated to a home five miles out of the city. There, the sickest child, who was to die within two months, was further isolated by being taken away from the other children and put with an adult case of pellagra in the last stages. Lavinder, who visited the orphanage in the summer of 1909, protested that isolation was unnecessary, expensive, and unwise, but protests were in vain. Tennessee began to isolate all its pellagra patients. The state board of health declared pellagra to be a transmissible disease and required physicians to report all cases.[65]

Fear of pellagra was probably worse in Tennessee than elsewhere. Exhibits on pellagra were prepared for the public, creating fear of the disease along with interest in it. Authorities first considered building a central hospital for the confinement of the pellagrous insane, then changed their tactic to urge all counties in the state to build isolation hospitals. Lavinder said that pellagraphobia originated in Tennessee and he hoped it would not spread very far.[66]

It did, in fact, spread beyond the bounds of the state. There was pressure for a quarantine in Kentucky, and pellagra patients at the Western Kentucky Asylum for the Insane were isolated. An informal isolation of pellagra patients was carried out at the Georgia State Sanitarium at Milledgeville, not because the physicians there thought the disease contagious, but rather because, as one doctor expressed it, these were "extremely filthy cases and . . . we put them there so they can be treated better." In Texas, a man with pellagra was actually isolated as a leper.[67]

Years later, it was observed that it was probably pellagra from which the Biblical Job suffered, not syphilis or leprosy.[68] Twentieth-century victims of pellagra in the American South well knew the anguish of Job, who, cast out on the village ash heap and shunned by his friends, cursed the day he had been born.

Isolation did not prevent spread of pellagra but instead heightened panic over it. Within two months after Tennessee built a house for the isolation of pellagrins, the state put a team of experts on pellagra in the field to allay the public's mounting fears. Meanwhile, the staff of City Hospital in Memphis found it utterly impracticable to carry out the isolation orders and finally succeeded in having the restriction lifted. Pellagrins were thereafter admitted to that hospital, and by 1914 the state board of health had rescinded its isolation order.[69]

Action taken by physicians at Memphis was the sort needed to curb pellagraphobia. At least part of the panic could be blamed on physicians, who, speaking hastily, made a deep and unfavorable impression on the already disturbed patient. To be told by the doctor, "Well, old fellow, you've got it" was enough to send one young man to the verge of suicide. Doctors were urged to be optimistic with these patients and to assure them that they need not be cast out from those they loved. Even if nothing could be done for the disease, something could be done for the patient. Significantly, the favorite prescription for "doing something for the patient" was to feed him well.[70]

Doctors blamed pellagraphobia on the press. If the press would stop printing such lurid details, saying that mortality from pellagra was greater than that from typhoid fever, there would not be such panic. One physician appealed to the South Carolina Press Association to print calmer accounts. Insanity generally attributed to pellagra was more often due to pellagraphobia, he maintained. The press resented the doctor's indictment. "It would be as just to blame the press for arousing apprehension at the discovery and announcement of any previously prevalent malady, be it diphtheria or typhoid fever or yellow fever," *The State* replied. "Unfortunately, only the fatal cases of pellagra are reported to the press. Consequently the public are informed only of the most serious cases."[71] *The State*'s righteous denial took no account of stories run recently in its own news columns in which pellagra was headlined as a "loathsome" or "dreadful" disease.

While fear still ran high, there were signs that in time a saner view would prevail. Both physicians and laymen began to look at the problem rather than to run from it. Pellagra was an issue in Georgia politics in 1911 when gubernatorial candidate Judge Richard B. Russell said he favored an appropriation for the state board of health to investigate the disease. In Atlanta, a pellagrasorium was opened in October 1911, the first hospital in the United States for treatment of the disease. Meanwhile, the Georgia Board of Health decided not to placard houses where pellagra patients lived. Such action had been contemplated. About the same time, officials of a mill in South Carolina requested aid from the Public Health Service in seeking the cause of pellagra in the mill community of Glendale. Mill authorities were understandably cautious and did not want anything to appear in public print about the investigation lest the people, who were inclined to be sensitive anyway, felt they were being used as guinea pigs. Besides, officials pointed out, it would not help business to have Glendale advertised as a pellagrous village. Officials of the Continental Coal Corporation in Kentucky were less reticent. They called a public conference, attended by physicians and laymen, to discuss the serious pellagra situation among its employees.[72]

Search for a pellagra cure led to a profusion of remedies, some logical, some unpleasant, some bizarre. More than two hundred, each one strongly endorsed, are recorded in the literature. The most widely accepted ones in the years immediately after the disease was recognized in the United States concentrated on diet, with emphasis placed on what foods to avoid rather than on what foods to eat. The success of a physician at the Georgia State Sanitarium in treating a pellagrin with raw eggs and milk seemed to attract little notice. Instead, some grocery stores capitalized on the great pellagra fear by advertising that they sold only pure foods, urging customers to shop with them and thus "keep off that awful disease pellagra." So few Jews had pellagra it was assumed they were immune. Jews credited their good fortune to the strict dietary rules of Leviticus and Deuteronomy. Corn, unknown to ancient Hebrews, was not a proscribed food, but Jews, especially Orthodox Jews, strictly interpreted the Mosaic law and ate only those foods which had the sanction of custom.[73]

Except as an adjunct to other treatment, however, the idea of a different kind of diet for pellagrins did not catch on. The most popular treatments, often touted and most discussed, were those using arsenic in one form or another. Arsenic had been used by the Italian Lombroso, and Americans accepted his proposed cure almost as quickly as they embraced the same professor's indictment of spoiled corn. Lombroso used an arsenic compound not because he thought it a true specific for pellagra, but rather because he considered it a valuable antidote for toxins of spoiled maize. He gave it by mouth in the form of Fowler's solution.[74]

Some American physicians, less cautious than Lombroso, adopted arsenic compounds not only as valuable antidotes but as specifics for pellagra. Some of the symptoms of the disease, especially the skin lesions and the nervous phenomena, looked somewhat like those of syphilis, so it seemed logical to use the same treatment. The fact that the Wassermann reaction of pellagra patients was nearly always negative was deemed unimportant to devotees of this theory. Arsenic was administered sometimes in the form of atoxyl, which was dangerous because an overdose could cause blindness, sometimes as salvarsan, popularly called 606, which caused chills, fevers, and occasional paroxysms.[75]

Treatment with salvarsan was long, expensive, and unpleasant. Six doses, given intravenously over a period of five weeks, were commonly recommended. The process should not be hurried, it was said, because pellagra organisms, "doubtless spirilla or spirochetes," were located in the nervous system and could not be reached readily by the circulating blood. They had to be killed gradually. The real problem with salvarsan was the severity of the reaction it sometimes caused. Salvarsan might send a pellagrin into spasms lasting six or eight days, leaving the already debilitated patient too weak to continue treatment. Supporters of salvarsan therapy, however, were not deterred by apparent failure. They thought it merely a matter of knowing how to use it properly, of regulating the dosage so that not too many germs would be killed at once. So confident was one doctor of the value of salvarsan that he charged his fellow physicians who refused to sanction use of the drug with letting their patients die.[76]

Salvarsan was tested at the Georgia State Sanitarium, where pellagra increased so rapidly from 1908 to 1912 that doctors tried almost anything to control it. Some of the patients showed marked improvement after treatment; others seemed better for a time but then relapsed. The final tally showed 18 percent recovered, 45 percent unimproved or relapsed, and 36 percent dead, hardly an impressive showing. Physicians there surmised that salvarsan's apparent beneficial effects were coincidental. They found the only constant factor in its use was the expense.[77]

The public was ready enough to accept salvarsan as a specific for pellagra. There were encouraging newspaper reports of its use in Georgia, Alabama, and North Carolina, and some people who had been caught up in the hysteria over the disease began to wonder how soon they could be cured with a single treatment of 606. The public enthusiasm was not shared by Lavinder who was even more disturbed over the use of salvarsan than he was over the attack on cottonseed oil. Salvarsan in pellagra, he wrote, "is not only useless but very often dangerous as well. To misuse a good thing and thus jeopardize its worth is an offense against common sense."[78]

Other drugs were tried, too. Calcium sulphide was used with apparent success in Wilmington, North Carolina. Dr. Charles T. Nesbitt, director of the Public Health Department there, was so impressed with results he wrote the Surgeon General about it. The method was "pure empiricism" with no scientific foundation for its use, but Nesbitt had the proof he wanted in the recovered pellagrins walking about the streets. Calcium sulphide was also endorsed by Atlanta's Mizell, originator of the cottonseed oil theory, who had gotten such prompt results that he felt like claiming it as a specific even without a knowledge of its chemical action.[79]

A Durham doctor recommended the clean-out, clean-up, keep clean treatment for pellagra to be achieved by large doses of castor oil every two hours. One in Louisiana treated all cases with quinine; another in South Carolina prescribed hydrogen dioxide to be taken internally followed by a tonic of iron, quinine, and strychnine. An unusual autoserotherapy treatment was used in Texas. A small square of cantharides plaster smeared with olive oil was put on the pellagrin's chest at bed time. A blister was raised by the next morning; serum was withdrawn from it and injected in the arm. This was repeated once a week. It was a treatment not unlike that commonly used three decades earlier for pneumonia.[80]

There was hope for several years that a serum would be developed for pellagra. This hope accounted for the interest in horses that recovered from the blind staggers, and occasionally, such an animal was offered to the Public Health Service. Transfusions of blood from recovered pellagrins were also tried in the hope that an antitoxin would be carried from one person to another. Doctors in Alabama tried transfusions using both cured pellagrins and healthy donors but with inconclusive results. Even surgery was recommended as a suitable treatment. In these cases an incision was made like that for an appendectomy. Instead of removing the appendix, however, the end was simply clipped off so that a syringe might be admitted and the bowel injected with a germicide.[81]

One of the most unusual treatments for pellagra used neither drugs nor serums but static electricity. A Florida practitioner seated his patient on an insulated platform, with his feet on a metal plate charged positively and his head covered by a crown electrode charged negatively. When the machine was turned on, there were roughly 200 discharges across the spark-gap per minute. Current traveled from feet to head and back again with every charge, vibrating every cell of the body and causing the patient's hair literally to stand on end. The cure worked, the doctor explained, because static electricity restored lost functions to atrophied brain and nerve cells.[82]

Patients who could afford it sought out the healing waters of mineral springs, and a positive cure was said to have been discovered in the medicinal waters at Mineral Wells, Texas. Fresh air, especially the cool air of the mountains, was deemed beneficial, and at least one attempt was made to provide cool air at home for a patient who could not travel. A New Orleans physician artificially refrigerated a room, which dropped the temperature by twelve degrees, for a pellagra patient. Doctors did not advise pellagrins to sun themselves, for patients nearly always got worse in sunshine and heat.[83]

There were many pellagrins, of course, who never consulted a doctor. These people relied on nature, home remedies, or pure luck to get them through an illness. Too poor to pay a doctor's fee and little inclined to seek professional help in any event, they formed a large potential market for patent medicines. Not long after it was definitely determined that pellagra existed in the United States, several "sure cures" for the disease, at least two purporting to be divinely inspired, could be found on store shelves.

"A wise Providence" was said to have handed down pellagra cures to businessmen in Alabama and South Carolina. The most spectacular quack was a mill worker in South Carolina with the unlikely name of Ezxba W. Dedmond who basked for a time in the glow of widespread public admiration. His product, "Ez-X-Ba River, the Stream of Life," sold for five dollars a bottle and was said to cure pellagra completely in a matter of weeks. Backed by substantial South Carolina businessmen, Dedmond launched his "cure" in 1911 when the wave of pellagraphobia was at the crest. A self-cured pellagrin, Dedmond claimed to be in partnership with God, who in His mercy, had shown him the remedy for the scourge. Huge advertisements were run in South Carolina newspapers proclaiming the marvelous curative powers of Ez-X-Ba River and extolling the generosity of Dedmond himself who offered to give away free bottles to the destitute.

An investigation of Dedmond and his remedy by the Public Health Service revealed many of the testimonials for Ez-X-Ba River to be fraudulent and the product to be worthless. Ez-X-Ba and a similar remedy called Pellagracide, prepared by another South Carolina firm, were exposed in *JAMA* in the spring of 1912. Not only was there nothing in them of curative value, but they tended to impair digestion. The situation, bad enough in itself, was aggravated by the fact that the products bore on their labels the statement, "Guaranteed under the Pure Food and Drug Act, June 30th, 1906." This led even the intelligent to believe that the government had control over such remedies.[84]

Pellagra was a social and a legal problem, as well as a medical one. Murders committed by people with advanced cases of pellagra were not uncommon, and occasionally a murderer was acquitted because of pellagrous insanity. Such was the case of a Chester, South Carolina, man who in 1913 shot a mill worker. The case created tremendous interest among medical men of the state because it hinged on the testimony of a physician that the defendant had pellagra and was insane. The next year another Chester man shot his neighbor in the head, a man with whom he had been most friendly. He, too, was found to have pellagra and was sent to the state hospital.

To the already knotty problem of pellagra was added the further complication of medical jurisprudence. Pellagra was a factor in criminal cases like those involving the two Chester men, where the tendency to homicide was irresistible, and it could be a factor in civil cases as well. The isolation in which pellagrins often lived, their melancholy ideas, religious fantasies, and delusions of persecution could affect their decisions. Any legal document a pellagrin signed, a will or a bill of sale, for example, could be contested later. But the line was a fine one; not every pellagrin was insane.[85]

Of more consequence than the occasional suicide or murder by a pellagrin was the tremendous weight that pellagra imposed on society. Like every other protracted illness, it posed social problems greater than death. The income of a family might be cut off for months or a year; the homemaker might be unable to look after her family; children might be kept from school. Both the family and society paid a heavy price. Pellagra and the social structure of the South were irrevocably entwined. Years before the definite cause of the disease was pinpointed, men of vision predicted that a social revolution would be required to wipe it out.[86]

2

Teamwork

BY 1912 THERE WAS a semblance of order in the search for the specific cause of pellagra. Two groups of workers were in the South that year systematically tracking down every clue. Armed with a healthy skepticism, these men were little inclined to take at face value everything the Italians had done. Instead, they gathered fresh data, cast out the old theories, and produced new ones of their own. The new team effort was conducted by the Public Health Service which began its pellagra work in a small way in 1909, and the Thompson–McFadden Commission, a privately endowed study conducted by the New York Graduate School of Medicine. Both groups observed the same phenomena, but there similarity in their work ended. They gave widely different interpretations to what they saw.

By coincidence Dr. Lavinder of the Public Health Service and Captain Joseph F. Siler of the Army Medical Corps, who was later to be a member of the Thompson–McFadden Commission's team, were in Italy at the same time during the summer of 1910, broadening their knowledge of the new scourge of the

South. Lavinder was traveling under orders from the Advisory Board of the Hygienic Laboratory, the research arm of the PHS. Captain Siler was working with Dr. Louis Sambon and the British Pellagra Investigation Committee. For a time, Lavinder traveled with this group; then they separated, each to go separate ways in Italy as they were later to go separate ways in America. Sambon was interested primarily in substantiating his theory that pellagra was caused by a parasite, and from his work that summer came his belief that the disease was borne by the simulium fly. Lavinder observed privately that Sambon's work was epidemiologic in character and uncontrolled by laboratory and experimental methods. He called it a "brilliant hypothesis," but that was all.[1]

Striking out on his own, Lavinder soon discovered that he had to get out into the country and visit peasants in the fields and in their homes if he was to see any pellagra cases. Few were to be found in the cities. He also visited the pellagra hospitals, and he called at the Bologna laboratory of Tizzoni who claimed to have discovered in *streptobacillus pellagrae* the true cause of the disease. At the time of Lavinder's visit, Tizzoni was using monkeys for his laboratory tests, but the American doctor observed that Tizzoni's monkeys seemed to be in perfect health. They showed no symptoms of pellagra.

When Lavinder came home from his European trip he was, in his own words, "on the fence." He had no evidence on which to base a sound conclusion as to the real nature of the disease, yet he doubted Sambon's hypothesis. He was not yet ready to discard the spoiled corn theory, yet it seemed the Italians were guilty of dogmatism. They could not think of pellagra except in terms of corn. If Lavinder and Captain Siler agreed on nothing else that summer, they agreed that the Italians were no longer studying pellagra; they were studying only corn. Both determined not to make the same mistake. Siler leaned toward the Sambon school, which sought the cause of pellagra in an insect; Lavinder had one foot in the camp of the Zeists who blamed pellagra on corn, spoiled or unspoiled, but he was unwilling to go all the way.[2]

One fresh idea came out of Lavinder's observations in Italy: he had to get patients and good laboratory facilities together. Perhaps remembering the two small rooms that had served inadequately as his laboratory at South Carolina's State Hospital for the Insane, he wrote from Italy that he wanted fresh cases brought to Washington for study. He suggested that this might be the first step in the establishment of a hospital in connection with the Hygienic Laboratory there.[3] The Pellagra Commission, appointed the year before by the Surgeon General, approved the idea and recommended that a twelve-bed hospital be established near the laboratory. Total expenses were estimated at $1,500 a month. If this were impossible, the commission proposed that a few pellagra patients be admitted for research purposes to one or more of the Marine hospitals. Since only seamen of the Merchant Marine could be treated in these hospitals, the latter course would require an act of Congress.[4]

Some action was imperative. Pellagraphobia was at its height throughout the South, and there were many calls for help. In Georgia, the state health board estimated that there were 50,000 cases in that state alone, a figure which medical men in other states said was probably far too high, but one which nevertheless had its influence with the edgy public when it appeared in the newspapers. Even church groups demanded action. The Baptist Tabernacle of Atlanta asked that a special commission be appointed to study the disease, and Georgia physicians and surgeons met to form an antipellagra association which planned to build a special hospital for the care of pellagra victims.[5] Babcock confirmed that pellagra had reached epidemic proportions in a broad belt across the South from Virginia to Texas. South Carolina's health director James A. Hayne was disturbed enough to discuss the situation with Congressman A. F. Lever, who asked that Public Health Service officers be sent into the state to investigate. The request was granted, and government investigators found the medical profession in South Carolina baffled and influential laymen worried. They realized that something ought to be done, but they were at a loss as to what to do. Surgeon General Walter Wyman in his annual report for 1911 said pellagra threatened to become a "national calamity." By 1912, more urgent calls for help came to the Public Health Service from Tennessee, where the number of cases had nearly doubled, and from Mississippi, where there were many counties with 50 to 150 cases each. North Carolinians were worried enough for Congressman John M. Faison to introduce a resolution in the House asking for an appropriation of $25,000 for the study of pellagra. State and provincial health officers at their annual meeting in 1912 asked the government to establish a commission to study pellagra.[6]

The response to these calls for help was swift. Congress approved the admission of pellagra patients to the Marine Hospital at Savannah, on the condition that only males in the early stages of the disease be admitted. Lavinder and an associate, Dr. R. M. Grimm, were sent to Savannah to work in the spring of 1911. Lavinder was to be in charge of the hospital; Grimm was to do the field work. A year later, help came from another quarter. Two Northern philanthropists, Colonel Robert M. Thompson of New York and J. H. McFadden of Philadelphia, donated $15,000 for a research expedition to make a study of pellagra in the United States. A three-man commission was appointed, including Captain Siler, Dr. P. E. Garrison of the United States Navy, and Dr. W. J. MacNeal of the New York Post Graduate Medical School. The Thompson–McFadden Commission planned to make an epidemiological study of an area in the South where pellagra was endemic, with necessary laboratory work being done in New York City. The commission set up field headquarters in Spartanburg, S.C., in June 1912.[7]

While the Thompson–McFadden Commission was being organized, a request was sent to the Public Health Service that Grimm be allowed to join it so that the Marine Hospital Service, as well as the Army and Navy Medical Corps, would be represented. The request was denied because Grimm was already deeply involved in the work at Savannah.[8] There were times in the months to come, however, when Grimm must have wished that he had been allowed to work with the commission. Its benefactors were generous; their $15,000 bequest sent the investigators off to their work well equipped; they even had an automobile. Compared with such affluence, the resources with which the government health workers had to work were slender indeed.

When Lavinder began his work in Savannah, he had no idea how long the job would take. He had orders to study the disease carefully, collect as many statistics as possible, equip a laboratory, and receive some patients for study. It required almost a year for the hospital to prepare for its first pellagrins—fourteen of them secured through advertisements in newspapers and medical journals. Most of them were not entirely suitable for the work that was planned, but Lavinder was not one to delay work because conditions were not perfect. He plunged ahead with clinical observations and laboratory work. His staff included, in addition to Grimm, a pharmacist, one nurse, and one laboratory attendant.[9]

The work at Savannah was difficult; Lavinder had to do his pellagra work as a sideline to running a busy hospital where there were as many as forty patients at a time. He did surgery, worked in the laboratory, and handled all the hospital's paper work as well. He even had to do much of his own typing on a machine which had to be coaxed, "cajoled along with gentleness," he put it. The laboratory equipment he needed did not arrive on time, and it usually cost more than the estimates. There was practically no library, not enough animals for his laboratory, and no really good place to keep those he had, since the hospital itself was located on half a city block. It was not easy to do research on a perplexing subject like pellagra under such conditions, but Lavinder was amiable and willing, and he did the best he could with the equipment and the staff available. His work and his spirits received a boost early in 1912 when he was relieved of all administrative duties at the hospital to devote all his time to pellagra studies. As a bonus, the staff at the Savannah hospital was increased, more books and equipment were secured, and more than twenty monkeys were sent from Washington for his laboratory.[10]

Still, there was never enough money for the work, "a fearful stringency in the government's finances," he told his friend Babcock. The matter of fifteen or twenty dollars for more laboratory rabbits was in the category of high finance. Worse than the shortage of funds was the perplexity of the problem and the seeming lack of progress in solving it. "I think I dream pellagra these days," Lavinder wrote Babcock, "but no inspiration comes to help me get a clue. The whole thing gets worse and worse to me." He said he went through about three phases a year on the etiology of pellagra, swinging wildly from Zeist to anti-Zeist and back again. It was "mental gymnastics with a vengeance."[11]

Meanwhile, the search for facts about pellagra began. The Department of Agriculture put two entomologists into the field in the spring of 1912 to investigate the possible relationship between insects and pellagra. These men were already at work in South Carolina when the team of investigators from the Thompson–McFadden Commission arrived in Spartanburg to begin their house-to-house check for pellagrins. By that time, Grimm had been in the field for almost a year investigating outbreaks of pellagra in South Carolina, Kentucky, and Georgia. Lavinder's clinical and laboratory work at the hospital in Savannah was important, but he thought that the work Grimm was doing in collecting statistics was even more vital. No one really knew how many cases of pellagra there were in the United States, and, until these cases could be located and the conditions around them studied, little progress could be made in solving the pellagra riddle.[12]

One of the places Grimm went seeking answers to his questions was Corbin, Kentucky. Within a radius of seven miles of Corbin, there had been fifty cases of pellagra in three years, with fifteen deaths and only two complete recoveries. The local medical association called a conference to investigate the "dread disease," as *The Louisville Times* headlined it, and Grimm was the chief witness. Later Grimm made epidemiological studies in South Carolina, working in the same area and at the same time as the government entomologists. To Lavinder's disappointment, Grimm and the entomologists had no instructions to coordinate their efforts, but worked independently.[13]

There were other problems that plagued Grimm's efforts in the field. He had to visit pellagra patients in their homes in order to see how they lived, and this was not always easy. Interviews could be conducted only when there was a local physician present, and doctors were often unwilling to spare the time. Once in the patient's home, there were further difficulties. The people were suspicious and disinclined to talk, and, when they did consent to an interview, their ignorance frequently made it impossible to obtain an accurate case history. Nor did Grimm have all the equipment he needed, and urgent requests were dispatched to Washington for such items as a camera and a traveling microscope. Travel, too, was complicated. He did not have permission to hire a carriage, and, unlike the team from the Thompson–McFadden Commission, was not provided with an automobile. A greater problem was monotony. Grimm told Lavinder he was discouraged in his work since case after case showed such sameness. "I am certainly at sea, but hope I am not aboard the Titanic," he wrote. Sunday was seldom a holiday for him. He visited pellagrins on Sundays, "substituting for other religious duties." Despite difficulties, however, Grimm's work was successful and it was important. His report gave urgently needed facts. Lavinder was delighted.[14]

Grimm's report was based on studies in twenty-five communities: three in Kentucky, seven in South Carolina, and fifteen in Georgia. In Kentucky, he visited the mountainous coal-mining district where houses were located around the mines or alongside creeks. He checked carefully the creekside houses because swift streams were the natural habitat of the simulium fly, the suspected insect carrier. He noted that the houses of the Kentucky coal miners were unscreened. Sanitation in these communities was almost uniformly bad, and typhoid was raging in one of them at the time of his visit. In Georgia, Grimm visited the homes of people he called typical "Georgia crackers," the sharecroppers and renters in rural areas and the mill workers who had moved to town hoping to find a better life. In South Carolina, he concentrated on the mill villages in the western part of the state, especially in the Spartanburg area where the county medical society promised him hearty cooperation. Many of the people living there had moved from the mountains of western North Carolina only to become sick shortly after arriving at their new homes. Grimm gathered information on many facets of life in the homes of pellagra patients. Some things the people told him in answer to questions; other things he merely observed.

It took no special wisdom to conclude that if there were an insect carrier for pellagra that there was ample opportunity for the disease to spread in all the areas Grimm visited. Bugs were there in abundance. Bedbugs were collected from several houses, and there was no reason to doubt they were present in many others. Houseflies were numerous; the buffalo gnat was often found; and corn, often as not, was infested with weevils and moths. Sanitary conditions left much to be desired. Water supplies everywhere were open to contamination, and facilities for the disposal of human waste were primitive or nonexistent.

Grimm checked on the food supply in pellagrous homes, too. He was not surprised to hear almost everybody say that they "had been raised on corn bread." Neither was it surprising to learn that much of the meal was made from "shipped in" corn which sometimes could be described only as "sorry." But there was more to the food supply than just corn, and Grimm opened a fertile field of investigation when he went beyond the matter of corn to question pellagrins on what else they ate and where they got it. This information was extremely difficult to obtain, for, as Grimm noted in his formal report, the memory and powers of observation of these people when questioned about their diet "seemed extremely defective." They were reticent to talk about a subject which spoke such volumes about their reduced economic status. He was able to find out that many people in the Southern pellagra districts lived almost entirely out of paper sacks. Few of them gardened. Most of their food was purchased from the company store or commissary, and in these stores the line of goods was meager, consisting primarily of dried or canned goods and packed meats. The physicians who visited these homes with him thought pellagrins were getting neither proper quality nor quantity of food, and they noted that it was poorly cooked. The South's reputation for fine cooking did not originate here. But since the food supply seemed equally limited and as poorly cooked in homes where there was no pellagra, no significance was attached to this observation. Everywhere he went, Grimm found pellagra patients living a hand-to-mouth existence. Their standard of living was for the most part "much below even a moderate standard." There were a few cases among the well-to-do, but usually pellagrins lived in an environment of poverty and bad hygiene.

The statistics Grimm gathered confirmed what others before him had observed: women were much more susceptible to pellagra than men. Of the cases on which he gathered data, more than 70 percent were females, with a ratio of white to Negro victims of almost six to one. If Negroes fell ill, however, they were much more likely to die than were white patients.

Grimm drew no definite conclusions on the cause of the disease, but he made some significant observations. Hard work and worry associated with the support of a large family seemed to pave the way for the development of pellagra. Poor living conditions and an insanitary environment were found so often in association with the disease that they could not be ignored.

Insects could be a factor, and there seemed to be some relationship between food and pellagra, but Grimm could not determine what it was. He suggested three possibilities: that food was a predisposing factor only, that certain foods actually were the real exciting agent, or that certain foods merely acted to exaggerate the symptoms. He observed that pellagra was much more prevalent than was ordinarily supposed even by physicians practicing in pellagrous communities, and he predicted that unraveling the etiology of this puzzling disease would be a "herculean task."[15] Although Grimm produced no answers, he did gather more concrete facts than anyone else had done before. The study of pellagra moved a step away from mere theorizing, a step nearer the scientific method.

Another Public Health Service officer noted a possible relationship between food and pellagra in 1912. Dr. B. S. Warren, assigned the duty of making a sanitary inspection of all the government buildings in Washington, D.C., every month, was sent to investigate the death from pellagra of an inmate at the government-operated Reform School for Girls. What he observed was significant, but little noticed, tucked away as it was in the *Annual Report of the Surgeon General*. "The sanitary conditions of the institution were found to be excellent, with the exception of the diet furnished to the inmates, which did not contain enough meat or other proteid element," Surgeon General Blue wrote. "Dr. Warren recommended that a better-balanced diet be furnished and records kept of the quantity given each inmate, together with the records of the weight and height of the inmates on admission and monthly afterwards, while the advisability was suggested of keeping records of hemoglobin percentage of the blood of the inmates."[16]

Meanwhile, the Thompson–McFadden Commission, in the summer of 1912, was making an intensive study of Spartanburg County, South Carolina. Their official report said this was done because a more intensive study of a small area would yield better results than a more superficial coverage of a large terri-

tory. There was also an excellent county map there showing
minute details, which the commission thought would be valuable.
This may have been only part of the reason why the commission
designed its study the way it did. The editor of *The Spartanburg
Herald,* Charles O. Hearon, commented some years later that,
when the Thompson–McFadden Commission came to the Pied-
mont to study pellagra, it was met with denials the disease existed in the principal towns. It was told it would not be welcomed, and the medical societies in those communities did not
offer to cooperate. In Spartanburg, it was a different story. The
commission worked through the Spartanburg County Medical
Society, and local doctors cooperated, in the words of the commission, "with alacrity." Wofford College offered the use of its
chemistry laboratory, and Babcock acceded to the commission's
request for autopsy material from the state hospital.[17] Led by
Siler and Garrison, the commission made maps of the terrain,
noted the location of houses, checked sanitation, cited the kind
of employment and the income of every family in the county,
searched for insect carriers, and investigated the food supply.

During the four-and-a-half months of their study (June 1
to October 15, 1912), the commission located 282 cases of pellagra in the county, or 35 cases for every 10,000 county inhabitants. It knew of 94 other cases, but these were not visited
because of early death or commitment to the state hospital. The
hardest hit districts were the cotton-mill villages where 104 of
every 10,000 people had pellagra. Whites were more often
affected than Negroes.

The commission sent fifteen pellagra patients from the county
to the headquarters in New York where the third member of
the team, Dr. MacNeal, supervised their treatment. They received no medicine during the acute stages of the attack, but
two were given arsenic after the acute stage had passed. Bacterial
and chemical studies were made, and it was observed that the
patient's ability to utilize various foodstuffs was only slightly
below normal. The workers in New York reached no conclusions.

The field workers in Spartanburg County reached no conclusions either. Women and children who stayed at home during the day were victims more often than any other group. About half the cases came from families with only one case and the rest from families with two or more. Except in the city of Spartanburg, which had a sewage system, sanitary facilities were poor. Houses were unscreened, and insects had free access to them. Working with the government entomologists, the commission investigated ticks, lice, bedbugs, cockroaches, horseflies, fleas, mosquitoes, buffalo gnats, houseflies, and stable flies. They ruled out everything but the housefly and the stable fly as possible carriers, even Sambon's favored buffalo gnat. If there were an insect carrier, the stable fly seemed the most likely offender.

The commission also observed that there appeared to be no difference in the diet of pellagrins and nonpellagrins. In Spartanburg County, the general diet of all the working classes was inadequate, especially in animal proteins. It could find no connection between corn and pellagra. Like Grimm, the commission observed that pellagra occurred predominantly among the poor. In 85 percent of the cases, the people lived on insufficient means. It noted that the income of mill workers, among whom pellagra was more prevalent than in any other group, was as low as 75¢ a day and the average was only $1.25.

Although Siler and Garrison, in their report of their first summer's work, carefully avoided drawing definite conclusions on what caused pellagra, they said that they regarded it as an infectious disease. It might be carried by the stable fly, although there was nothing definite to point to this, or it might be an intestinal infection transmitted by contaminated food.[18]

A week or so before the Thompson–McFadden Commission completed its first year's field work, the second national meeting on pellagra was held at Columbia. Like the first conference, this session was held at the State Hospital for the Insane. Unlike the earlier conference, however, there was little said at this meeting about corn. In 1912, the emphasis shifted to the germ theory.

There was nothing concrete to connect pellagra with germs, but there was some circumstantial evidence. Pellagra was often found where there was poor sanitation. It seemed as logical to connect the disease with this fact as it had three years earlier to associate it solely with corn. The shift of opinion in 1912 was strongly toward the anti-Zeists.

Resolutions adopted by the conference carefully avoided the issue of what caused pellagra. These recommended that measures be taken to prevent the sale and consumption of spoiled corn, not because this product had been found guilty, but simply because it had been incriminated. Conference delegates also resolved that pellagra was not transmissible from man to man and that quarantine and isolation measures were unnecessary and unwise. This resolution was not passed without argument, however. MacNeal of the Thompson–McFadden Commission tried to get it amended so that it would include the possibility of pellagra's being transmitted by insects or other media.

The conference was attended by some 150 people, less than half the number who had come for the first pellagra conference in 1909. But among them was Surgeon General Rupert Blue, a native South Carolinian who only recently had assumed his duties as the nation's chief health officer. The invitation to Blue was extended by Babcock through Senator Tillman. Blue was impressed by the meeting, calling it an "epoch-making" gathering of scientists banded together to seek the solution of a problem of national and international importance. He called on the general public to urge lawmakers to appropriate money for pellagra work. "It is a rather sad commentary on our business astuteness that we have failed to recognize the economic importance of protecting the public health," he said. The conference elected Lavinder as president of the National Association for the Study of Pellagra and expressed the hope that Congress would appropriate funds to maintain a national body to do research.[19]

In his annual report for that year, Blue noted that pellagra occurred primarily in well-defined endemic areas: "Whether these areas are determined by the topography, the flora, the fauna, climatic conditions or the special manner of life, or customs of the inhabitants remains to be determined, and when this has been done the discovery of the cause of the disease will without doubt be near at hand."[20] While it may have seemed obvious to Blue that the disease was concentrated in a well-defined area, there were those in the South who hailed with satisfaction the appearance of pellagra in other sections of the country. *The State* noted editorially during the conference that it had been proved that pellagra exists in all parts of the United States: "Possibly it may be more common in one part of the country than in others, but it is well established that it is not a local disease and that it is not confined to one class of citizens." A few days later *The State* twitted the *New York Times* for erroneously describing pellagra as an aftereffect of hookworm infection: "Now that physicians in the north are belatedly recognizing the existence of pellagra in that section, and the disease has therefore come to have local news interest, New York newspapers would do well to recommend their copyreaders to the medical dictionaries."[21] The South Carolina press deemphasized the peculiar significance of pellagra in the South in other ways, too. In contrast to 1909, when the gathering of medical men to study pellagra was the biggest news story for several days, the conference in 1912 was accorded but little space. Small things in themselves, the skimpy coverage given the conference and the barbed editorial comments were harbingers of a changing attitude toward pellagra in the South. Early panic was being replaced by pride. Pellagra was not a very nice thing to have. If the South could not wish it away, it would take what comfort it could in appearance of the disease in other regions of the country.

In the light of what the years to come were to reveal about the nature of the disease, there was one very important paper read at the meeting of the National Association for the Study of Pellagra in 1912. This was by the Englishman Dr. F. M.

Sandwith, who had suspected that pellagra existed in the United States for years before the first case was reported. Using a new approach, Sandwith asked if pellagra might be due to a deficiency in nutrition. He based his inquiry on the monumental work of Sir F. Gowland Hopkins who, in 1906, had discovered that rats and mice needed something in their diets which he called an "accessory food factor." Dr. Hopkins had found that young mice fed a diet in which the only nitrogenous constituent came from zein (*zea mays*) did not grow well. When tryptophane, an amino acid absent from the decomposition products of zein, was added, they grew much better. In rats, the missing quantity was supplied in but two cubic centimeters of milk a day. Sandwith suggested that pellagra might be but an outward indication that some specific "hormone" or other substance essential to the processes of the body was missing.[22] This was a theme Babcock advanced in one of the discussion periods at the conference. He made an analogy between beriberi, sprue, scurvy, and pellagra. If there were a dietary deficiency in pellagra, then such a deficiency would affect any debilitated patient whether the debility was caused by tuberculosis, insanity, alcohol, or syphilis.[23]

But American students of the disease, leaning toward acceptance of the germ theory of pellagra, paid little attention. Meanwhile, Dr. Casimir Funk, working in a London laboratory, returned to Hopkins's work with the "accessory food factor." Funk had coined a new word, "vitamine," for the mysterious missing quantity. He believed this to be a chemical amine, a term which he then combined with the Latin word for life. Funk suspected that pellagra, like beriberi, was caused by a lack in the diet. Fifteen years earlier, it had been proved that a diet of polished rice led to beriberi; whole grain rice prevented it. He thought that modern milling methods, which stripped off the outer layers and the germ of the corn kernel, might be responsible for robbing corn of its nutritive value and consequently might be the real cause of pellagra.[24] In the United

States, Funk's work was accorded no special significance, although Carl Alsberg of the United States Department of Agriculture did examine maize to see if it contained any of the same chemical substances found in rice polishings.[25]

The faulty-diet theory was appealing although it was not taken seriously. "How gladly would we if we could say that this disease was due to some particular form of diet alone," South Carolina's health officer Hayne told other state and provincial health officers at their meeting in 1912. "Then our task as a Board of Health would be comparatively easy!" Hayne thought it carried by an insect.[26]

The Thompson–McFadden Commission returned to the field in 1913, taking up its intensive investigation of the Spartanburg area, looking primarily for a source of infection. Its main departure from the pattern of work in 1912 was to set up a charity hospital in the Spartan Mills village in a building provided by the mill owner. The main thrust of their work, however, continued to be an intensive epidemiological study. They visited the home of every mill worker in six mill villages in Spartanburg County and made a complete record of everything that might conceivably have any connection with pellagra. They marked the location of the house and the length of time the people lived there, and they recorded the sex, age, occupation, and relationship of every resident. They also took a case history of every pellagrin, including "a very complete record of his diet." The commission was interested especially in the possible influence of foods on pellagra and on the location of the domicile of those who already had the disease to the domicile of those who later developed it.[27]

In the midst of their work in the summer of 1913, the prestige and morale of the commission were bolstered by a personal visit from the famous Dr. Sambon of London, who had been decorated by the King of Italy and accorded worldwide fame for his successful work with tropical diseases. The Thompson–McFadden Commission called a special conference in Spartanburg to hear Sambon speak. He expressed great appreciation for all the work being done in the United States on pellagra, especially that being done by the commission. Interviewed in New York, Sambon said that food had absolutely nothing to do with pellagra, that everyone at the Spartanburg conference had agreed that it was an infectious disease carried by an insect. He himself thought it was the buffalo gnat; the government entomologist thought it was the stable fly.[28] That was of no matter. What was important in Sambon's view was that the maize theory had been exploded.

The results of the commission's elaborately planned study apparently did rule out all connection of food with pellagra. They had made careful inquiries about the use of all corn products, including cornmeal, grits, syrup, and corn whiskey. They concentrated most of their attention on the two kinds of cornmeal, imported and local, for meal was the most universally used food. More than half the families ate shipped cornmeal every day, and it was this group that had the least pellagra. The disease occurred most frequently among those who never used shipped cornmeal. Local cornmeal was rarely used, and the commission could find no connection between it and pellagra. The daily use of fresh meat was found to be rather uncommon among the residents of mill villages, and, in four of the six villages surveyed, fresh meat was available at the local markets only during the colder seasons of the year. But, according to the commission's findings, those who never ate fresh meat at all were the least likely to have pellagra. The only food that seemed to have any connection with pellagra was milk. The disease was less common among those families who used it daily.

All the evidence the Thompson–McFadden Commission gathered seemed to point to the fact that pellagra was in some way related to the place where the victim lived. They found most pellagra patients either in the same house with another victim or living next door or across the street from one. They concluded that pellagra spread in a community from a preexisting case as a center, but that it spread readily only within a very·small area surrounding that case.[29]

Having ruled out diet altogether, the commission narrowed its research to a possible insect carrier. By 1913, the stable fly like the simulium fly was ruled out. The commission now thought the housefly, the louse, or the bedbug a more likely carrier.[30] In any event, it held that the real root of the pellagra problem lay in poor sewage disposal. Neither in the rural areas of Spartanburg County nor in the mill villages were sanitary facilities adequate. The commission members drew maps of Spartanburg on which they located the sewer mains and the houses in which all pellagrins lived. They observed that pellagra occurred where the sewer mains stopped. They compared the unsewered mill villages of Spartanburg County with mill villages like Newry in other parts of the state which had had water-carriage systems for years. In Newry there was no pellagra; in Spartanburg County villages, it was rife. The commission concluded that pellagra might be an intestinal infection transmitted by contaminated food. At any rate, it was a theory worthy of further study.[31]

The Thompson–McFadden Commission received support for its views from the National Pellagra Commission, established in 1910 by the all-Negro National Medical Association. Negro doctors, denied membership in white medical associations in the South as part of the developing pattern of segregation after 1890, formed their own association in 1895. In a drive to improve the health of the Negro people, the NMA created three commissions in 1910 to deal with health problems particularly affecting them. There was one for tuberculosis, one for hookworm, and another for pellagra. The latter commission was headed by Dr. A. M. Townsend of Nashville, Tennessee, who was credited with recognizing the first case of pellagra in Nashville. Townsend's group said that only an insect carrier could account for the spread of the disease across the country "like a prairie fire." They cited no specific carrier but expressed the conviction that pellagra must be transmitted in much the same way as malaria and yellow fever.[32]

There were others, however, including officers of the Public Health Service, who seriously doubted the validity of the Thompson–McFadden findings. *The Journal of the American Medical Association* cautioned against accepting the theory. It was based solely on epidemiological studies, *JAMA* pointed out, and, in working with diseases of unknown origins, these were not always to be trusted. There was no reliable means of distinguishing essentials from nonessentials. What appeared trivial might well be of great importance; and, conversely, what appeared to be of importance might ultimately prove to be negligible.[33]

The Public Health Service launched an ambitious program of pellagra investigations in 1913. Fortified by a budget of $45,000, almost a quarter of the entire $200,000 appropriation for public health, Lavinder and his associates intended to confirm or disprove the infectious character of pellagra. They could conduct feeding experiments using monkeys and chickens, make bacteriologic studies in the laboratories, conduct epidemiologic studies in several Southern states, and try new treatments on patients in hospitals. Tryptophan, the amino acid which Sir F. Gowland Hopkins had found was essential to proper growth of mice, was cited specifically as one thing which would be tested. Basic to all these studies was the collection of statistics. A special effort would be made to find out just how many people had pellagra.[34]

Earlier efforts to collect statistics had been somewhat haphazard. A postcard survey in 1912 of 18,000 physicians in eight Southern states—Virginia, North Carolina, South Carolina, Georgia, Kentucky, Alabama, Mississippi, and Louisiana—had yielded fewer than 5,000 replies. At first Lavinder believed this meant simply that a physician had no cases to report; later he decided this meant rather a large number of unreported cases. A few months later, he rounded out his study with a survey of Arkansas, Oklahoma, and Texas. In all, he found 19,915 reported cases of pellagra in the South from 1907 to 1912, with a mortality of 40 percent. According to these findings, women pellagrins outnumbered men by almost three to one, and whites outnumbered blacks by the same ratio. Lavinder's map showing the area in which pellagra was prevalent looked like one of the Confederacy with Kentucky and a corner of Missouri added.[35]

The situation was so serious in Mississippi in the summer of 1913 that the state board of health asked Lavinder to personally investigate. For the first time, a special effort was made to get really accurate statistics on the prevalence of pellagra. The results showed what had not been apparent before: blacks seemed to be as susceptible to pellagra as whites. They had just not been counted before. In the first six months of 1913, there were 1,313 cases of pellagra in Mississippi, more than half of them among Negroes. There were 268 deaths.[36] The rich delta region between the Yazoo and the Mississippi rivers was most affected. There, Negroes predominated in the population about ten to one. Lavinder found little pellagra in Jackson or Vicksburg, noting that "pellagra is not an urban disease." Lavinder thought that all the farmers there, white and Negro, looked well fed and prosperous. He noted that they were fairly well housed, but that surrounding hygienic conditions were like those usually found in the Southern states, that is, objectionable. Diet of the Negroes was abundant and varied, he wrote. "It consists largely of corn bread, molasses and salt meat. But this is supplemented by fish, which are abundant in the streams, game at times, and fresh garden truck during the summer months." He observed that Negroes ate the cheapest grade of meal and that their molasses probably contained corn syrup. Curiously, Italians living in the area, a people so often accused of bringing pellagra with them on the boat, were free of the disease.

While in the Mississippi area, Lavinder conceived the idea

for his next large research project. In New Orleans, he visited the Tulane University laboratory of Dr. W. H. Harris, who had reported the successful reproduction of pellagra in the rhesus monkey from the injection of material from a pellagrin. At the time of Lavinder's visit, the only surviving monkey had recovered, but Lavinder thought the results of Harris's work were suggestive enough to demand further study.[37] Returning east, he went straight to work. In August 1913, Lavinder and Grimm, joined later by two other doctors from the Public Health Service, Edward Francis and W. F. Lorenz, began extensive work with monkeys. They used seventy-seven rhesus monkeys, two Java monkeys, and three female baboons and tried by every means possible to infect them with pellagra. They used injections, suspensions, extracts, and emulsions, all without success. Eight monkeys died, four with diseases that definitely were not pellagra, the other four from undetermined causes.[38] This was not Lavinder's first effort to transmit pellagra to monkeys. He had failed in 1911, too, the same year that two of his associates at the Hygienic Laboratory reported a similar failure. One of these was Dr. Joseph Goldberger, whose name after 1914 would loom larger than any other in pellagra investigations. After Lavinder's second unsuccessful attempt to induce pellagra in monkeys, his attitude toward all those who said that it could be done was one of "frank agnosticism."[39]

The failure of the monkey experiments pointed the work of the Public Health Service in another direction. If the disease were not infectious, it must be connected with metabolism, and, for metabolic studies, a special hospital was necessary. There was already sentiment and some pressure to build a government pellagra hospital somewhere in the South so that proper experimental work could be conducted and clinical observations made. Lavinder had looked for a suitable building while in Mississippi but had found none.

South Carolina Congressman Joseph T. Johnson was anxious that the proposed hospital be located in his state. He introduced a bill in the House to authorize the Public Health Service to acquire a site near Spartanburg and build a hospital for the investigation and treatment of diseases, especially pellagra. He asked that $300,000 be appropriated.[40] This was a staggering sum in light of the fact that the previous Congress had appropriated to the PHS only $200,000 to investigate the disease of man and the pollution of water supplies. The bill did not receive support. The Treasury Department was skeptical of embarking on a policy of building hospitals in individual states for the treatment and study of a particular disease for fear the Public Health Service might be led beyond the well-established lines of its work. Surgeon General Rupert Blue was wary, too. He knew that more intensive work needed to be done in the Spartanburg area, but not on the grand scale that Congressman Johnson proposed.[41]

The initiative for establishing a government pellagra hospital in Spartanburg came largely from local leadership, although Senator Tillman was working behind the scenes. The Senator warned Babcock against getting the state board of health involved lest it create the impression there was a concerted movement to induce national authorities to work in South Carolina, thus making other states jealous enough to block the game. Tillman was working in concert with Congressman Johnson. It was before Senator Tillman, Congressman Johnson, and Surgeon General Blue that a committee of Spartanburg citizens appeared in 1913 to ask for the hospital. Funds for the Thompson–McFadden Commission had been curtailed and the Spartanburg committee—composed of the editor of the newspaper, a banker, and a local physician—wanted the government to continue the work of the commission. Editor Charles Hearon of the *Spartanburg Herald* remarked years later that, in 1914, although the spread of the disease was appalling, "no community was willing to admit the seriousness of the situation until Spartanburg citizens came to the front to request the government to take a hand to determine its origin and provide a cure."[42]

Spread of the disease was indeed appalling, but as a matter of fact a kind of inertia toward the pellagra problem began to settle over the South by 1913. Spartanburg was one of the few areas which did not fall victim to it. *The Southern Medical Journal* urged states to cooperate in the pellagra investigation and asked doctors to organize efforts in each locality. "Wake up, brothers, to your opportunities and your duties!" the *Journal* editor said in the summer of 1913, but not very many were listening.[43]

The quest of the Spartanburg delegation was successful. In mid-December 1913, the advisory board of the Hygienic Laboratory recommended that a temporary hospital and laboratory facility be established in the South. If diet were a factor in pellagra, every article of food under suspicion would have to be tested. Highly technical chemical and metabolic studies were necessary, studies which could not be conducted at the Marine Hospital in Savannah. The board estimated the cost of operating the hospital for one year at $47,000. The Secretary of the Treasury, in requesting funds from Congress, based the appeal on the grounds of both health and economics. Several important industries were implicated. It was important to determine once and for all what bearing, if any, foods had on the continuance of pellagra.[44] Congress passed the emergency appropriation, and the Pellagra Hospital was opened in Spartanburg in June 1914. It occupied the same building in Spartan Mills village which the Thompson–McFadden Commission had used the year before for charity pellagra patients.[45]

With approval given for the Pellagra Hospital, the Public Health Service was ready to submit the corn theory of pellagra to the most extensive tests ever conducted. It would begin afresh the search for toxic substances in corn products and through these, if any were found, try to produce symptoms of pellagra in animals. Special dietary studies were conducted among the patients admitted to the hospital. Several different diets were tried, ranging from all vegetable to all meat, and elaborate tests were set up to determine the exact effect which these had on the patients. The function of kidneys and liver was tested, records of blood pressure and body weight were kept, and stomach examinations were made frequently. The work was difficult, for the patients were uninterested in the experiments and, being pellagrins, could seldom remember, much less follow, instructions.[46]

While PHS officers worked in Spartanburg to try to find exactly what pellagra did to the body, a young Wisconsin psychiatrist began work at the Georgia State Sanitarium at Milledgeville to try to discover exactly what it did to the mind. He was Dr. William F. Lorenz of the Wisconsin State Hospital, who was appointed to a temporary position on the PHS staff, and had earlier worked with Lavinder and Francis in the monkey experiment. Since 1911 the trustees of the sanitarium had urged the PHS to send someone to Milledgeville to study pellagra, but it was not until the pellagra work was greatly expanded that the invitation could be accepted. By 1914 when Lorenz arrived, the need for help at the Georgia State Sanitarium was acute. There was a "remarkable increase" in the number of pellagra patients that year—a total of 365 cases. Of these, 190 died. That was slightly more than one death from pellagra every other day for the whole year.[47]

Lorenz spent seven months in Milledgeville making his tests and observations. He was joined about midway in the project by PHS officer Dr. D. G. Willets, who was sent to assist in the investigation. They had complete control over two wards of female pellagra patients and access to all of the hospital's departments and records. There were enough cases of pellagra in the hospital to allow them to observe its mental manifestations in many stages, from hallucinations to apathy. Lorenz concluded that pellagra could bring out a latent mental disturbance and that the pellagrous psychosis was similar to that of acute alcoholism. He suggested that the disease might be caused by a toxic substance with a chemical nature not unlike alcohol.[48]

Knowledge about pellagra was accumulating. Americans were beginning to write books about the new disease, which had appeared so mysteriously in the South. Three had been published by 1913. The first of these, published in 1910, was a translation by Babcock and Lavinder of the French physician A. Marie's *Pellagra,* which was itself an abridgement of Cesare Lombroso's monumental work. It included a prefatory note by Lombroso written just before his death, as well as Babcock's and Lavinder's own pertinent observations. The translator–authors, while proud of their work, were sorry when it was done that they had not written their own book throughout. "We could have made a better book with less work," Lavinder confided to Babcock, "and it makes me angry to think that Marie's name must be put on what he deserves no credit for whatever. Confound him anyway. Your remark that he would do well now to retranslate the book into French expresses the thing exactly."[49]

Two other books were published by 1913, both by Atlanta physicians, George M. Niles and Stewart R. Roberts, which helped fill in the rather wide gap in the pellagra literature, for relatively little had been written in English, but they did not provide any fresh insights into the problems involved.[50] More valuable was the work of the Public Health Service, which pointed to a toxic substance, perhaps in food, as the most likely cause of pellagra, and the Thompson–McFadden Commission, whose work led to the belief it was caused by an infection. The picture of the disease they hoped to construct was taking shape, but it was far from complete. Their work raised almost as many questions as it answered. Why were women affected so much more often than men? Could Negroes be as subject to the disease as whites?[51] Was pellagra inheritable? Was it rural or urban? Were altitude and topography factors? The studies gave conflicting answers. There was no answer supported by convincing proof to the one big question about pellagra: What caused it? This one loomed as large as ever.

3

Meat, Meal, and Molasses: An Indictment

THE ANSWERS to some of the questions about pellagra came with dramatic swiftness in 1914. No one expected results so soon, but even before the government's Pellagra Hospital opened in South Carolina, the riddle was on its way to solution. The key was found on the kitchen tables of the South: people had pellagra because they did not eat well. This observation, simple enough in itself, opened the way through scientific mishmash to a deep, fruitful channel of research, which, in the next quarter of a century, yielded answers to seemingly unanswerable questions.

This turn in the course of pellagra investigations came when the Public Health Service decided to give the problem more support and attention. Forty-one men were put in the field to study pellagra from every conceivable angle and their work was financed with the comparatively large sum of $80,000 for the first year. More important, when Lavinder requested other work, Surgeon General Rupert Blue appointed in his place Dr. Joseph Goldberger. From that day in February 1914, Goldberger's name and pellagra were inseparably linked.[1] Goldberger brought the light of a perceptive mind to the problem, which, as it unfolded, brought him both endless satisfaction and a large measure of frustration. In time, it also brought fame.

Goldberger was a big man, six feet or more, and red-headed, with piercing eyes which looked straight through rimless glasses. At first glance he seemed to be cold, rigid, and incapable of emotion. There were those who thought him cynical, a man lacking faith or even interest in humanity. But these were people who did not know him well. With his family and his associates, he was warm and compassionate, a person capable of experiencing great joy or crushing disappointment. His published writings were coldly precise, and his official memorandums and reports to the Surgeon General gave no hint that warm blood coursed in his veins, but letters to his wife and children revealed a man with a big heart. When his pellagra work went well in the South, when those who once seemed hopelessly ill began to get well, he wrote his wife, "They are all well!!!"[2] It was more than a mere expression of satisfaction with his work.

Goldberger was a Jewish immigrant. Born on a farm in Hungary in 1874, he was seven years old when his parents brought him to America. They settled in New York City's East Side, where the older Goldbergers ran a small grocery store for which Joseph and his brothers served as delivery boys. He made rapid progress in school and was an avid reader, enjoying especially Horatio Alger stories and the high adventure of James Fenimore Cooper. Mathematics was his favorite subject, however, and at sixteen he entered the City College of New York to study civil engineering. At the end of his second year he stood fifth in his class of 600. Then by chance, he accompanied a friend to a lecture at the Bellevue Hospital Medical College and decided immediately that he was in the wrong field; it was medicine he must study. He dropped civil engineering and entered Bellevue Hospital College from which he was graduated with honors in 1895. He served his internship and engaged in private practice for two years, but gave this up because it was not very exciting and besides, he did not like to send out bills. When the Spanish-American War broke out, he thought about joining the Navy Medical Corps and was one of 2,000 applicants applying for 40 vacancies. The navy never ordered him to appear for examination. The next year he took the examination for a commission in the Marine Hospital Service and made the highest score. As a Public Health Service officer (the name was changed in 1902), the only bills that burdened him were those he had to pay out of a slender salary, and he found excitement enough.

His first assignment was as an immigration officer at Ellis Island, New York, and later at Reedy Island, Philadelphia, but in 1902, anxious for some excitement, he went to Washington and begged to be allowed to work on yellow fever, then endemic in Tampico, Mexico. His request granted, Goldberger went to both Mexico and Cuba and had his work well underway when he fell victim to yellow fever himself. There were some advantages to this misfortune. On his recovery, now immune to the disease, he could pursue the work in earnest. Moving to Puerto Rico, he raised mosquitoes and studied them in order to learn how they might be more easily eradicated. Among other things, he found out a mosquito could travel only seventy-five yards on its own, but could move long distances on railway cars. His detailed article on yellow fever, including a long discussion on the anatomy of mosquitoes, so impressed his superiors in Washington that Dr. M. J. Rosenau, director of the PHS's Hygienic Laboratory, invited Goldberger to join his small staff.

The Hygienic Laboratory was the research arm of the Public Health Service, an expansion of the bacteriological laboratory established by Dr. Joseph J. Kinyoun in 1887 in one room of the Marine Hospital on Staten Island and a forerunner of the National Institutes of Health. The laboratory was moved to Washington in 1892, and became the Hygienic Laboratory in 1902, the same year the Marine Hospital Service added "and Public Health" to its name. Its principal duties at first were to secure the effectiveness of various serums and vaccines, but it soon branched out into other areas of research. An advisory board, composed of some of the nation's leading scientists, was appointed the first year of the Hygienic Laboratory's existence, and two years later the laboratory moved into a new building occupying a five-acre site on the Naval Observatory grounds.[3] Director Rosenau set high standards for his staff. "Everybody is expected to do intelligent and faithful work," he told them the first day they moved into the new building. "The cooperation of all is needed. . . . If anything goes wrong every one is to feel at perfect liberty to tell the Director who will endeavor to properly administer justice." All officers at the laboratory, as in the rest of the Public Health Service, held rank and title comparable to those of the military—surgeon, assistant surgeon, passed assistant surgeon—and they had special rules to follow. Muster was held every Saturday morning at ten o'clock when the particular part of the building, the grounds, and the work assigned to each one was inspected. Rosenau warned his staff from the first against extravagance. Bills for running the laboratory amounted to $50,000 a year, he said, "from which it is evident we must keep down expenses and exercise economy wherever possible." He also admonished them to do nothing to irritate or aggravate the navy, whose grounds the laboratory occupied, to be kind to animals with which they worked, and to be extremely careful always: "We deal with the most virulent infections known to man."[4]

In his early years at the laboratory, Goldberger had reason to remember Rosenau's caution against infection. Yellow fever was not the only disease he contracted in the course of duty. In 1907 while working with dengue fever in Brownsville, Texas, he became a victim himself, and in 1910, after having been bitten by a body louse in Mexico City, he developed a severe case of typhus fever. In his work on typhus, he confirmed the French scientist Nicolle's idea that it was spread by a louse, proved that this disease and Rocky Mountain spotted fever were distinct diseases, and discovered that Brill's disease, prevalent in many American cities, was really a mild form of typhus.

He enjoyed working in the field, and his approach to any new problem was thorough. Investigating a typhoid fever epidemic in Washington, D.C., in 1906, he made a meticulous survey of the entire Potomac River, field experience that proved invaluable in the later pellagra studies. A few years later, he was called to Philadelphia to investigate an outbreak of a sudden epidemic of a strange and disabling rash called straw itch or Stramberg's disease. A large number of sailors and some hotel employees were affected. All were poor, all recovered on being admitted to the hospital, and all had just acquired new straw mattresses. Goldberger thrust his arm into one of the mattresses and had three volunteers sleep on them. They all developed a rash and itch. Sifting through the straw and looking at it carefully through a hand lens, Goldberger soon found the small insect responsible, the Acarina mite. It had taken but forty-eight hours to solve the case. More important was his work on measles, part of a long process that eventually led to the elimination of that disease as a serious threat to health. He had turned his attention to diphtheria and was at work on an epidemic in Detroit when Surgeon General Blue put him in charge of the pellagra investigations.

The rapid increase of pellagra in the South made it one of the nation's most serious health problems, one which called for the greatest skill the Public Health Service could command. Goldberger's expertise in working with infectious diseases earned him the new assignment. "I feel that you are preeminently fitted for this work and it could be placed in no better hands," Surgeon General Blue wrote him.[5] Goldberger did not want the job and faced it with the greatest reluctance. Certainly the new work meant another long separation from his family, and he suspected that it might be a waste of time. After his first trip through the South, however, where he inspected the problem at first hand, his initial depression gave way to eager acceptance of a challenge. He was never discouraged again. After only three weeks in the field, Goldberger saw what others before him had merely looked at without really seeing. The clue to pellagra was in the monotonous three-M diet of the poor of the South: meat (fatback), meal, and molasses. Goldberger returned to his Washington headquarters in buoyant spirits, ready to begin work on a problem on which he would spend the rest of his life. His wife could see the "light of battle in his eyes."[6]

On that first field trip through the South, Goldberger did his work almost entirely by observation. With the all-encompassing eye of the civil engineer he might have been, he looked beyond the pellagrins themselves to the way in which they lived in the boxlike houses of mill villages or on tenant farms where cotton grew up to the doorstep and where there were few gardens and almost no cows in sight. He saw what the poor ate, corn bread, fatback, and syrup at almost every meal, and he noted that the well-to-do, the only group which as a class was free from pellagra, were not subjected to such dietary monotony. Being an outsider was an advantage to him. Meat, meal, and molasses looked very strange to him and so took on a significance which those who had seen it every day of their lives missed.

The popular three-M diet had deep roots. It dated from frontier times when meat was an important item in the diet and when the abundance of wild game made it easy to obtain. As towns and villages moved westward and game became scarcer, the frontiersman turned to salted meat easily provided by pork. The pig became a fixture; it ran free in the woods and it thrived on easily grown corn. The grain that fattened the pig also provided meal, the second staple in the diet. The third, molasses or syrup, was quickly made from cane which grew as readily as corn. This diet became the staple for slaves on Southern plantations and for the common white man as well. The transition from frontiersman to cotton farmer was too gradual to cause a break in food habits.[7]

Insofar as convenience was concerned, the diet of meat, meal, and molasses was ideal for the land of cotton. The immense amount of hand labor in planting, chopping, and picking cotton left little time for growing food crops. The one-horse cotton farmer had to get along on the most efficient foods he could get, and salt pork, cornmeal, and syrup were, if nothing else, efficient.[8] They were easy to procure, easy to keep, easy to cook, cheap, filling, and reasonably tasty. When the one-horse farmer lost his independence and became a tenant, he did not change his diet. Indeed, the old dietary staples of the frontier proved to be a great boon to the plantation owner who furnished tenants with food. Nothing could be so easily handled in the plantation commissary or in the company store of the mill village.

On his Southern tour, Goldberger visited the Public Health Service Laboratory at Savannah where the monkey experiments were underway, and he observed that not only did the monkeys seem to be quite well but so did the men working with them. Not even Edward Francis, who caught every disease he ever worked with, was ill. How could pellagra be contagious?

Goldberger made mental notes of all he saw. Exactly three weeks after he accepted his new assignment with such misgiving, he submitted a memorandum to the Surgeon General, which completely revamped the pellagra investigation and set it on a course which was to yield fruitful results. He wanted the monkey experiments to continue so that this aspect of the etiology of pellagra could be disposed of once and for all. He wanted work Dr. Lorenz had begun at Milledgeville on the psychiatric aspects of pellagra to be continued, and he suggested other studies be conducted there as well. He wanted geographical studies of pellagra resumed on more intensive lines. More important, he planned extensive studies on diet to find out what effect a new diet might have in insitutions like asylums and orphanages where pellagra was endemic. He suggested that experimental diet studies, including extensive metabolic tests, be carried out in the new hospital in Spartanburg as planned.[9]

In the next few months he made repeated trips throughout the South visiting asylums and other institutions in Georgia, Alabama, Florida, Kentucky, and Mississippi. Everywhere, he just looked and listened. He carried no monkeys or rabbits with him. He set up no laboratories; he carried no microscope. Unencumbered by equipment and preconceived ideas, he brought to the two-centuries-old pellagra problem a fresh perspective and a new approach. By late June 1914, after less than five months on his new assignment, he announced that a faulty diet caused pellagra. In a short article in *Public Health Reports* he urged people to reduce the cereal content of their diet and to eat more fresh meat, milk, and eggs. It was too good news to keep to himself.[10]

This advice was based primarily on his observations at Georgia State Sanitarium at Milledgeville, the first institution selected for the new studies. At Milledgeville, his attention was attracted first to pellagra patients, of whom there were several hundred at the time of his first visit. Next he looked at the nurses and attendants who spent a large part of every day in the wards. Curiously, none of them was ill. He followed them about their work at the hospital wards and went with them to the dining room at mealtime. It was there that he made a very important observation. He had been told that inmates and attendants ate the same food, that they were served from the same kitchen, even out of the same dishes. But Goldberger quickly saw that this was not strictly true. There was a difference in the diet of the inmates and the patients. The nurses and attendants always served themselves first, selecting the best and the greatest variety, giving the patients what was left. In addition, they had opportunity to supplement their diet elsewhere. The inmates did not.

There was ample written evidence testifying to the inadequacy of the diet at the Georgia State Sanitarium. In 1910, four years before Goldberger made his first visit to Milledgeville, a legislative committee investigated the hospital and made inquiries, among other things, about the food. From the testimony of both inmates and attendants, an account of mealtime horror could be pieced together. The food supplies were skimpy. Breakfast consisted of grits, beef hash, biscuits, and coffee. For dinner, there was a small piece of boiled beef a couple of inches long and an inch-and-a-half wide and some vegetables cooked, some patients said, like "hog slop." There was less for supper—just light bread and syrup. No buttermilk was served; only occasionally was there sweet milk for the patients, but the attendants drank it twice every day. One inmate said he did not get enough to eat to feed "a good hungry mockingbird." Another said it would be better to hang than to starve.[11]

Inmates had to "scuffle" to get enough to eat unless they happened to be one of the "star" boarders or pets who always got the best pieces of meat. Patients who were not petted and those who lacked sufficient drive to piece out a meager meal went hungry. The easiest way to get more food was simply to steal something off somebody else's plate, and this was often done. Apathetic patients, and there were many of these, suffered most. Doctors seldom came to the dining room to see that patients were fed properly, and attendants paid them little attention. Some patients testified that there was always milk on the attendants' table, that they had "nice meat and hash," but that if a patient went around to ask for anything "they snatch you up quick as lightning."[12]

Hearty fare could hardly have been provided on the slender resources with which the hospital had to work. The total operating budget for the hospital in 1910, including salaries, medicine, supplies, and maintenance, was only thirty-four-and-a-half cents per patient per day.[13] In good years, the food supplies of the hospital were augmented with vegetables, meat, and milk from the hospital farm and garden. Much of the 3,000 acre farm, however, was used for growing cotton and corn, which were sold and the proceeds put into the general hospital fund. Many years, too, the garden was not a success. Nearly every year the superintendent of the hospital had to report that the garden had not prospered, that there had been too much rain or not enough. One year the hogs on the farm died of cholera; the next, thieves stole the little pigs. In 1913, the year before Goldberger came, the oat crop was good, but unfortunately, that was the year officials had decided to reduce the acreage planted in oats. Meanwhile, the trees in the orchard yielded little fruit, and it was too dry for good pastures, so the amount of milk from the dairy was less than it might have been.[14]

In the hospital dining rooms, Goldberger noted the amount and quality of food eaten, and he observed that it was from the cases of terminal dementia praecox and other apathetic types that the other patients stole food. These people, so timid that they often hid in nooks and corners of the hospital, made no effort to defend their rights in the dining room. If all but the gravy were snatched off their plates by hungry neighbors, they made no protest. Unless such patients were carefully supervised, Goldberger pointed out to his associate, Dr. Lorenz, they were very apt to receive an inadequate diet over a long period.

Goldberger's plan of work for the hospital grew directly out of his observations in the dining room. He suggested that Lorenz give the twenty-seven acute cases of pellagra, which were under his care, a diet that more nearly resembled that of well-to-do people. It included at least a half pound of fresh beef a day, several eggs, green vegetables, and milk. Seven of the patients died, and the condition of three remained unchanged, but thirteen others improved, and four were designated recoveries. Considering the class of patients with which he was dealing, Goldberger found the results "notably favorable." When Lorenz's work at the hospital was complete, two women's wards, one for white patients and the other for Negroes, were turned over to Goldberger for his study. To each one of these were admitted forty patients who had had pellagra attacks during 1914. To insure that most of these patients would remain in the hospital under observation for at least a year, he selected for the test

only those of a "much deteriorated, untidy class." Diet therapy
was begun in the fall of 1914 under the direction of Dr. David
G. Willets, whom the PHS had sent down the previous spring
to assist Lorenz.[15]

Meanwhile, Goldberger had found two orphanages in Jackson,
Mississippi, which agreed to cooperate in the government's study
of pellagra. At the Methodist Orphanage in Jackson there were
68 orphans out of 211 (32 percent of the total) who had pellagra
on July 1, 1914. At the Baptist Orphanage a half-mile away,
the situation was even worse. In a population of 226 children,
there were 136 positive cases and 24 suspected cases. Nearly
all of the victims were between six and twelve years of age.
At the Methodist Orphanage, only 2 children under six had
pellagra; only 1 over twelve was affected.[16] This curious exemption of the little children and those over twelve was comparable
to the exemption of the attendants and nurses at the Georgia
asylum. Goldberger could explain it only in terms of diet. The
little ones had some milk every day; the older ones, many of
whom had some work to do around the orphange, were given
more lean meat and other animal protein food.

Goldberger was horrified at what he saw. At the Baptist Orphanage, 60 percent of the children had pellagra in the spring
of 1914. "But," he wrote his wife, "if one excludes those of
the children whose work or duties give them extra food the
percentage goes up so frightfully high that I don't dare to name
it." The children were given such a poor diet that he thought
a little muckraking would not hurt. Indeed, it was his opinion
that they were not fed as well as cattle. He recorded their diet
of the previous winter.

6:30 A.M. *Breakfast:* Grits, gravy, biscuit and syrup.

12N. *Lunch:* one roll.

3 P.M. *Dinner:* Vegetable soup, boiled vegetables: turnips, cabbage,
sweet potatoes, corn bread, syrup or molasses.

Some pork once a week—Sunday dinner.[17]

He noted that not one matron had the disease; they were distinctly better fed than the children.

The experiment for the orphanages was much like that for the asylum. Goldberger proposed to supplement the diet at these children's homes with meat, milk and dried legumes. The constant association of pellagra with starchy foods very strongly suggested to him that the disease was in some way dependent on a faulty diet. He did not know exactly what the fault was, but it was one that was either prevented or corrected by the addition of larger proportions of protein.[18] At Milledgeville, he hoped to cure pellagra by dietary means; in Mississippi, he hoped to prevent it. He estimated that it would cost $700 a month at each orphanage to buy the necessary food.[19] Beginning in September 1914, the government paid this bill for the next two years.

Very early in his work in Mississippi, Goldberger decided that pellagra might possibly be prevented by a protein less expensive and more readily attainable than meat, eggs, and milk. Perhaps the answer to the problem lay in the very simple and cheap matter of beans. He wrote confidentially to his wife that "it seems probable that pellagra can be wiped out in our South by simply getting the people to eat beans, Beans, BEAns, BEANs, and BEANS!!! If they will eat enough 'flageolets' they can eat anything else they D—please." He was not quite sure of this, but if it proved true, he thought it would be a "very great strike."[20] A few days later he observed that "BEANS" were looking up. If Southerners would only eat those legumes in the winter, he thought pellagra would dissipate like a mist before the sun. He wanted Southerners to eat beans the year round.[21]

Certainly, he encouraged the children at the Methodist and Baptist orphanages to eat beans. In the new government-sponsored diet they were served beans every day. The new diet also included fresh meat three or four times a week and milk twice a day for the children aged six to twelve, and three times a day for those under six. There were eggs every morning for those under twelve; oatmeal replaced grits for breakfast. Corn bread was served just once a week. Goldberger changed nothing at the orphanages but the diet. Both institutions were over-crowded and they remained that way. In both, the hygienic and sanitary conditions "left much to be desired." He deliber-ately left these unchanged. If there was a reduction in the inci-dence of pellagra, then diet alone could be singled out as being responsible. Whether or not the diet would prevent pellagra, it made Goldberger a popular man at the orphanages. Children gathered around to thank him for the good food. They hoped it would not stop.[22] The local press printed Goldberger's ideas about diet and pellagra, giving them the prominence of a two-column headline, and the state board of health distributed copies of his dietary proposals to all county health officers and heads of institutions in the state. Dr. C. H. Waring, left in charge of work at the orphanages, was shortly invited to address a meeting of local physicians on the "live and timely topic" of pellagra.[23]

A year after the diet-supplement plan began at Methodist and Baptist orphanages in Jackson, success of the program was marked, and officials at Baptist Orphanage acknowledged their indebtedness to the Public Health Service. The annual report of the orphanage described the health of the children as being better than it had been for years, and praised the PHS for its work. There can be no doubt that the cause of pellagra is dietary, the report continued, and in the future, management at the home could control the situation. "We are profoundly grateful to the Public Health Service . . . for the faithful and helpful service rendered in our time of need and we most heartily commend their treatment to all who suffer from pellagra."[24] That very month, however, at Methodist Orphanage a half-mile away, the superintendent was issuing his annual plea to the citizens of Mississippi to send carloads of goods to the children's home for Thanksgiving. Both Jackson orphanages depended on this annual gift to help make ends meet. The message of diet apparently had not fallen on very receptive ears at the Methodist institution, however, for the superintendent in asking for food requested people to send "molasses, corn, flour, sugar, grits, cured meats, all kinds of canned goods."[25] There was not a request for foods that would prevent pellagra—not even beans—or for money to buy them.

Meanwhile, Goldberger continued his constant round of visits throughout the South with occasional quick trips into the North. The more he saw, the more convinced he became that his diet theory was correct. He visited an insane asylum in Philadelphia. "Curious!" he noted. "There was not a case of pellagra there."[26] He saw many pellagrins who appeared to be well nourished, so he knew that pellagra was not a starvation disease in the ordinary sense of the word. It was a strange hunger, an under-nourishment or starvation in a sense hardly dreamed of before.

Casimir Funk had suggested that pellagra was a vitamin deficiency disease caused by overmilled corn, and one of Goldberger's associates in the Public Health Service, Dr. Carl Voegtlin, agreed that pellagra and vitamins were linked. At the University of Wisconsin, a famous experiment with cows fed on a single-plant source had shown that something was missing from certain monotonous diets, and, two years before Goldberger began his work on pellagra, a young biochemist at Wisconsin, Elmer V. McCollum, had discovered the first vitamin, fat-soluble A. For a time, Goldberger thought pellagra might be caused by the presence of excessive amounts of some poison like soluble aluminum salts in the vegetable component of the diet rather than by a lack of something, but he never doubted that the problem could be solved by adding better quality protein. He was sure that experiments at Milledgeville would prove him right, but his sense of social duty would not let him wait a full year to announce publicly a theory he was certain was correct, one, admirable in its simplicity, which could prevent thousands of people from becoming ill.

At orphanages a modification of the diet alone was enough to prevent pellagra, he said. At asylums the problem was more difficult, for there it was necessary to see that the patients actually ate the food they needed. Serving it was not enough. He estimated that at least half the pellagra cases occurring outside the institutions could be prevented if the people actually ate the diet that was available to them, but that, for a margin of safety, they should eat fewer starches and more proteins.

Goldberger's theory fitted neatly into the whole pellagra picture. It provided answers to heretofore unanswerable questions. It explained why the disease always appeared in the spring rather than at other seasons of the year. "Pellagra is a sort of spring crop following a lean winter diet," Goldberger said.[27] It explained why pellagra was so intimately associated with poverty. When income was low, people skimped on their diet, eliminating expensive items like milk and meat and subsisting on cheaper items like fatback, meal, and molasses. It also explained why the poor of the South had been afflicted rather than the equally poor people of the North. There, even among the poor, the diet was much less starchy. Hookworm might be partly responsible for this, Goldberger said. It perverted tastes from foods which people should eat. There was even an explanation of why this disease of the poor appeared occasionally among the well-to-do. He blamed these cases entirely on eccentricities in taste.[28]

Food was the answer to the pellagra riddle. Goldberger was sure of it. He quoted the French physician Theophile Roussel who in 1866 had written that "without dietetic measures *all remedies fail*."[29] This explained the reports of success with the disease following doses of arsenic, for the treatment was nearly always accompanied by a modification in diet. What pleased Goldberger most about the new theory was that it released the South from the grip of fear. There was no basis in fact for pellagraphobia.

The association of diet with pellagra seemed so obvious to Goldberger that he had difficulty understanding those doctors who had successfully treated pellagra by dietary means and yet saw no connection between the two. At the Baptist Orphanage in Hapeville, Georgia, the diet was modified (for no apparent reason) a full year before Goldberger began his work at the orphanages in Mississippi. Dramatically, the number of cases of pellagra dropped from sixty-four to zero. When Goldberger visited there in September 1914, he was excited, for here was advance proof that his diet therapy projects would work. At the same time he was amazed that the Georgia doctor who had changed the diet could not see the success of his experiment. "[He] is as blind as a bat; he doesn't see a thing—no light to him, at all," Goldberger wrote. "Indeed it is nothing less than wonderful that a thing so striking, so notable means so little to him, has so little significance for him."[30]

Whether the board of trustees at the Georgia State Sanitarium knew the significance of what it was doing, it gave Goldberger and Willets a free hand and full cooperation in the studies they had underway there. The doctors not only had complete control over two wards, but they were free to make recommendations which applied to the institution as a whole. This they did. Willets assured the superintendent that the ration then issued by the institution was considered sufficient to prevent the development of pellagra, but that special care must be taken to see that the timid, withdrawn patients ate their share. He recommended that indifferent or slow eaters be fed in separate groups and given more time for their meals. Nurses and attendants should have different meal hours from the patients, and they should have a somewhat better diet from that of the inmates so that they would not be tempted to take for themselves the best portions of the food.[31]

In the PHS wards the diet was greatly modified. Patients were served fresh milk for breakfast, buttermilk for lunch and dinner, a half-pound of fresh beef a day, and a serving of the much-favored dried beans or peas. Some patients improved so rapidly under the regimen that they were released from the hospital before the year's study was complete, but seventy-two remained under observation for almost a year, or at least until the anniversary date of their last attack. Not one showed any sign of pellagra.[32]

This success with food was all the more dramatic when contrasted with the appalling situation in the rest of the hospital and in the South at large in 1915. The incidence of pellagra at Milledgeville reached a new peak. that year. There were 433 cases and 220 deaths. This was 35 percent of all the deaths in the institution, or 3 deaths every 5 days.[33] For the first time, the annual report of the sanitarium mentioned food in connection with pellagra. The government experts "do not seem to have lost faith in their theory that the cause of the disease is due to improper diet," the superintendent noted. The government experts were, in fact, so sure that they were correct that late in the year they added another 50 patients to the ones they already had under observation.[34] The results in Mississippi were even more successful than those in Milledgeville. The children who the year before had been listless and marked with the ugly red splotches of pellagra showed the bloom of health in the spring of 1915. There was not a single case of pellagra at Methodist Orphanage and only one recurrence at the Baptist Orphanage.[35]

The successful experiment at the orphanages in Mississippi was repeated the following year in South Carolina. Goldberger had hoped to begin work at the Epworth Orphanage in Columbia late in 1914, but the doctor there was not interested in cooperating, so the project was dropped for a year. The doctor, Goldberger said confidentially, was "a plodder without the right sort of training and equipment and not quite big enough to realize it and so give another man a chance."[36] In late summer, 1915, however, Goldberger had his chance. He began the same diet routine that he followed in Mississippi and with the same successful results.

This is "no flash in the pan," Goldberger told the press when he arrived in Columbia. The diet therapy at Epworth Orphanage was to be continued for a year or two. "Naturally, it is going to cost the government some money, but it shows when we agree to furnish part of the diet necessary for the treatment of pellagrins how thoroughly we are convinced that the disease is brought on solely by improper dieting and because we are positive that with a well-balanced diet pellagra can be absolutely done away with."[37] The caution to be careful with the government's money had apparently taken firm root.

The conditions at Epworth Orphanage were, if anything, even worse than those in Mississippi. There were 245 children there, 150 of whom had pellagra one or more times before 1915. The children ate in two dining rooms—the younger children in one and the older children in another. Of the younger children, more than 88 percent had pellagra; 41 percent of the older children were also affected. The diet at the orphanage was meager indeed. There was no meat except for bacon boiled with the vegetables, which little children did not like, and a skimpy 40 pounds of beef, which was stretched out each week among the entire population of the home. Larger girls who helped in the kitchen appropriated some extra food for themselves and their friends; boys who did the milking were known to drink some before it was delivered to the kitchen. For the others, the quantity of meat per child per day was less than one and one-eleventh ounce, and three-fourths of this was salt pork. A third of a pint of milk a day for each child for all purposes was described as an "outside figure." The crop of beans and peas had been short, and no extra food was ever purchased when the population of the orphanage increased.[38]

Goldberger found all the children well when he checked them in the spring after he began the supplementary feeding program. In August, when the work at the orphanage was finished, the children were absolutely free of pellagra for the first time since the discovery of the disease there in 1908. As he surveyed the place on leaving, Goldberger had, as he put it, a "grippy, 'thrilly' feeling. . . . The most skeptical must and will be impressed."[39]

But not all the skeptical were impressed. In fact, as soon as the PHS completed its test program at the three orphanages in September 1916, one of them returned immediately to the unmodified and unsupplemented institution diet. Within a few months, 40 percent of the children again had pellagra. When, under Goldberger's direction, the diet was once more supplemented with meat and milk, pellagra vanished.[40]

Goldberger might have expected this reaction, but apparently he did not. The plea from Methodist Orphanage the year before for more grits, flour, and cornmeal, while the diet-supplement program was still underway, was a portent of things to come. The dietary habits of generations were not to be changed easily, and the desire to cut corners and save money was strong. With outside financial help, a health program might be possible, even attractive. Without such help, the picture was different. Not even the antihookworm campaign was maintained at full level after the Rockefeller money was exhausted in 1914. Successful as that program had been, some states cut back or abandoned their programs of hookworm eradication when left on their own financial resources. Georgia, for example, entirely abandoned its hookworm work after the commission withdrew.[41] If there was sagging interest in the relatively simple problem of hookworm disease, where the cause was definitely known and could be seen under a microscope, and the cure—at least a temporary one—cost only about fifty cents per person, how difficult the problem of maintaining an interest in the dietary cause of pellagra would be.

Meanwhile, work was still underway at Savannah where pellagra patients were being treated at the Marine Hospital. The program of clinical observation which Lavinder began there in 1912 when the first patients answered his newspaper advertisements continued until September 1915, when all clinical work was moved to the Pellagra Hospital in Spartanburg. There were some dramatic recoveries at the Savannah hospital where the sole treatment consisted of a diet rich in milk, fresh meat, eggs, and dried beans. The hospital also tested some tonics and medicines, including the much-favored Fowler's solution. Most of the patients who took these improved, but so did those who took only a placebo, as well as those who received nothing at all. Questioned about what they had eaten for the three months before entering the hospital, the patients at Savannah reported a diet consisting mainly of biscuits, corn bread, syrup, white meat, or sowbelly. Nearly three-fourths ate no beef whatever; only half ate eggs. A few raised chickens at home, but they sold the eggs rather than use them on the family table.[42]

At Spartanburg, the work of the Pellagra Hospital was expanded to include an outpatient clinic, an unusual one that dispensed no medicine at all, only food. The patients, all with moderately severe cases, came to the clinic every day for dinner. Some continued to work in the nearby mill and children continued to go to school. The clinic, another of Goldberger's ideas, opened November 1, 1914, and stayed open until the hospital itself was closed in 1920. The average patient recovered fully in from six to ten weeks, and there was no recurrence of the disease among those who came to dinner even after pellagrous symptoms had disappeared. Occasionally, a person would be discharged as cured, only to be readmitted again a few months later after prolonged exposure to home cooking.[43]

Another aspect of the program at Spartanburg, one that was to assume a major role by 1916, was a systematic probe into pellagra's relation to poverty. Economic conditions were obviously connected with the disease, but the exact relationship was not clear. It was fairly easy to note that a vegetable diet was usually cheaper than one containing meat and that people of meager means would thus depend more on vegetable and cereal foods. It was far more difficult to prove that this was, in fact, true and that there was a direct correlation between this and pellagra. There was little specific information on the economic, sanitary, and dietary conditions prevailing in communities where pellagra was prevalent, and it was extremely difficult to obtain.

Carl Voegtlin, a PHS pharmacologist working in the Spartanburg area, commented to the home office in Washington just
how difficult his task was. He found mill people to be suspicious
of any stranger who entered their house and tried to get information about the way they lived.[44] A complicating factor was the
pellagrins' deficient mental state. They could not be depended
on to answer questions correctly even if they consented to answer
them at all.

An early devotee to the theory of a vitamin deficiency as
the cause of pellagra, Voegtlin needed exact information on
what pellagrins had eaten before they became ill. As a start
he went with Dr. Garrison of the Thompson–McFadden Commission to check the quality of food sold at the store in Inman
Mills village where the workers usually shopped twice a month.
Looking at the order books, Voegtlin was surprised to find such
monotony in the diet of the people. He was especially shocked
by the absence of fresh meat except during the few cold weather
months from November to February. One family in the space
of a month in the spring of 1911 bought a hundred pounds
of flour, a half bushel of meal, some lard, salt pork, and "preparation," the name given alum baking powder. The only variety
the diet afforded was one can of peaches, one of salmon, a
nickel's worth of crackers, and a jar of pickles. Three members
of this family soon had pellagra.[45]

A year after Goldberger began his pellagra work, he was invited to give the Cutter lecture on preventive medicine at Harvard University. The invitation surprised him, and he was at
first tempted to decline, for he had so much field work underway
that he did not want to divert his attention to something he
considered "essentially frivolous."[46] He accepted the invitation,
however, and lectured on pellagra and diet. The same spring
he received other invitations to lecture on the same subject,
some of which he declined. He was not quite far enough along
on the research to give too many lectures, and, furthermore,
the people who attended the lectures were not the ones he

wanted to reach. He was much more interested in reaching those who lived on bread and molasses and who had pellagra than he was in lecturing to the "silk-stockings" who were interested in the subject only to the extent of discussing it over their beefsteaks.[47]

He had already granted some newspaper interviews to spread his favorite gospel of beans. "To cure pellagra eat beans," he said. "To prevent pellagra eat more beans." By the summer of 1915 he expanded his advice to those Southerners who had pellagra or who seemed likely to get it. "Own and care for a cow," he said. Nothing was more important than a good supply of milk. Diversification of crops was second in importance only to this. He advised all tenant farmers to plant a five-acre patch in cowpeas or field peas, and he urged landowners to set aside acreage for peas instead of planting it all in cotton. His pamphlet on the prevention of pellagra was widely distributed by state health departments to small towns and farming communities throughout the South; 80,000 copies of it were distributed in Georgia alone.[48]

Goldberger never doubted the rightness of his cause. By the summer of 1915 he was convinced that his work would be a "mile-stone in the history of preventive medicine." He was excited over the marvelous possibility of so easily saving thousands of lives and of preventing the misery of years of ill health and suffering. To him, it seemed possible that with enough nourishing food he could bring the dead to life.[49]

Some doctors hooted at Goldberger's diet theory soon after he announced it in 1914, still claiming that pellagra was an infection. At the meeting of the Southern Medical Association in Richmond in 1914 Goldberger got a taste of things to come. James A. Hayne, South Carolina's health officer who would become Goldberger's most vocal opponent, called the "recently promulgated bean theory . . . an absurdity." As far as reaching a solution to the cause of pellagra, we seem to be as far away from it as ever, he said.[50] The discussion continued long after the SMA meeting was over. In Louisiana, the issue of what caused pellagra was a lively one. The minister of the First Baptist Church in Shreveport pronounced solemnly from the pulpit, "no one knows the cause of pellagra." Doctors of the state were inclined to agree with him. State health officer G. C. Chandler, who believed the disease to be communicable, was afraid to put the public in the "fanciful security" of the government's theory. After a stormy all-day session of the Louisiana State Board of Health, in which the doctors failed to agree on anything, not even the pronunciation of the word, the board tentatively accepted the PHS view that pellagra was not communicable, but they were not convinced about the decision.[51]

Goldberger attended the SMA meeting in Richmond and the session of the Louisiana State Board of Health, in both places defending the diet theory. While calm in public, privately he hooted at the scoffers: "They are thrown into a state of mental fog and confusion if you cannot instantly explain every reported epidemiological observation," he confided to his wife. "They reason that inasmuch as I cannot instantly explain every observation that therefore, I must be wrong. It never seems to occur to them that the observation they want explained may be erroneous."[52] He was pleased a few months later when some of the doubters began to agree with him. Dr. Babcock seemed convinced, as did a leading Memphis physician and the state health officer of North Carolina. Mississippi's health officials were "sold" on diet. "Without any other successful line of treatment for pellagra," health officer Galloway said, "it is the duty of every physician to follow the suggestion of Dr. Goldberger in the treatment of pellagra." Goldberger thought results of his work should convince all those with "sound minds." "Let the 'heathen' rage!" he said.[53]

There were few "heathen" at the third triennial meeting of the Association for the Study of Pellagra in Columbia, South Carolina, in mid-October 1915. Goldberger, making his first appearance at one of these sessions, reported the success of supplementary diet programs at Milledgeville and the Jackson orphanages. Claude Lavinder, president of the association and Goldberger's associate at the Public Health Service, was worried about the paper's reception, but afterward congratulated Goldberger on "putting it across."[54]

This conference, like the earlier ones, was held at the State Hospital for the Insane, but there had been some important changes at the hospital since the 1912 meeting. Babcock had resigned as superintendent in 1914 amidst a blaze of publicity and a legislative investigation of his institution. Among other things, Babcock was accused of having brought injury to the reputation and progress of South Carolina by calling attention to the prevalence of pellagra in the state. The investigation exonerated Babcock completely of any wrongdoing. Problems of the hospital were instead blamed on serious understaffing, too little money, and too much politics.[55] Babcock returned to the hospital to attend the pellagra conference and took an active part. Fewer papers were presented at this meeting than at the others, but, as the local press observed, they represented more research. There was less emphasis on theory and more stress on facts, facts which the association decided would be wise to share with Negroes since blacks as well as whites had pellagra. Black physicians were invited to sit in the gallery.[56]

Goldberger's paper was not scheduled until the second day of the conference which opened with a "remarkable" evening session at which Siler, Garrison, and MacNeal of the Thompson–McFadden Commission reported on work they had been conducting in Jamaica and Barbados. As soon as they had finished, Goldberger opened the discussion with a criticism of the statistical methods used by the commission. The reaction to his criticism was lively. Many doctors present said they had never encountered such interest at a medical convention. The meeting began at 8:30 P.M. and did not conclude until 1:30 A.M., when Lavinder adjourned it over shouts of protest. One doctor who left early and retired, on hearing of the discussion, got up, dressed, and returned to the floor to make a speech. Another came back to make "a splendid argument."[57]

The discussion brought out once again the age-old argument on what caused pellagra. Was it a faulty diet or was it some germ? Was diet a predisposing factor or the only essential factor? The doctors reached no conclusion that night. Babcock summed up the evening's discussion well when he compared exposition of all the different theories to the "Eight Blind Men of Hindoostan" who described the elephant. One felt the tail and pronounced the elephant to be like a rope; another the ears and concluded the beast to be very much like a fan; the third a leg, and said the animal must surely be like a tree. Each was partly right, yet all were wrong. "We should study the problem of pellagra with humility," Babcock said.[58]

Delegates to the conference received a surprise next morning. On the front page of the morning paper was a story datelined Washington, D.C., which, without a trace of humility, announced proof of the dietary cure for pellagra. Without mentioning Goldberger by name, the PHS reported the successful treatment of the disease by diet alone in Georgia and Mississippi. The story linked pellagra with the deteriorating economic status of Southern wage earners, particularly in the cotton goods and lumber industries. Since the industrial depression of 1907, a PHS spokesman said, wages had been lower, and retail prices of food had been higher, particularly in the South. The increase had been at least 40 percent higher in proteins than in carbohydrates or hydrocarbons. Southern wage earners, with a lessened financial ability to provide a balanced diet, were victims of pellagra more often then ever.[59] Estimates of 1,000 cases of pellagra in the South in 1909 were deemed hazardous; in 1915, 75,000 was a reasonably safe estimate.

That same morning Goldberger, with his associates Waring from the orphanages and Willets from the Georgia hospital, formally presented the paper that had already been reported in the press. Goldberger was happy with its reception. " 'Diet' wins by a large majority," he wrote home. The enemy had "half owned up in public meeting." The "enemy" included supporters of the infection theory like South Carolina's health officer Hayne who withdrew his own paper and "bleated very gently" when his time to speak came around, and Captain Siler of the Thompson–McFadden Commission who stated on the floor he agreed with everything in Goldberger's paper and later congratulated him personally. "Siler is a gentleman," Goldberger commented.[60]

Goldberger was probably not a very good reporter. If he had listened carefully he would have heard something more than a "bleat" from Hayne. Scheduled to speak on the "communicability of pellagra," Hayne did withdraw his paper saying he would wait to talk about that until someone could show the real bacillus. But he did not stop there. He was glib, angry, and probably a bit more than worried. The general practitioner has his problem solved, Hayne admitted. The treatment for pellagra was diet. But what about the man who is charged with preventing disease? What about the public health officer?

Apparently forgetting completely that only three years before he had wished that pellagra were caused by a faulty diet for then the problem would be so easy to solve, he now found a dietary solution to the problem fraught with difficulties: "When you tell the health officer that the way to stop this thing is to make the whole people of the state change their mode of living, you put a proposition up to him that is almost impossible." The health officer would prefer dealing with something he is accustomed to, Hayne said, namely communicable diseases, for then he knows how to handle the situation. Where does one start on a disease due to economic conditions existing in the South?[61]

Hayne made a good point. It was indeed difficult to change a mode of life. Nevertheless, Goldberger thought the diet "bandwagon" would rapidly fill and that it would not be long before there was a general squabble on who saw it first. The conference left open the road to acceptance of the dietary theory. For the first time, it passed no resolution on the cause of pellagra. In 1909 and again in 1912, there had been resolutions on this facet of the study, even if they were expressed in negative terms only. At the 1915 session, the resolutions were merely expressions of thanks. This might have been all that was possible. Members of the resolutions committee represented three distinct schools of thought: Goldberger of the dietary school; Siler, spokesman for infectionists (at least until he heard Goldberger's paper); and J. J. Watson of South Carolina, champion of the once-popular spoiled corn theory.[62]

If the conference avoided the issue of what caused pellagra, the local press seemed ready enough to accept Goldberger's ideas. *The State* called his paper "remarkable." "While the knowledge which underlies the diet theory may not be new, the Public Health Service certainly deserves high credit for having made use of this knowledge in such a practical manner as well as in teaching a distressed population a feasible method of solving their difficulties. Some of the greatest discoveries in the history of medicine are not really discoveries but practical applications of previously known truths."[63]

While Goldberger achieved a seeming victory at Columbia, the timing of the meeting was actually unfortunate for his purposes. It came just ten days before the end of his most famous and controversial research project, the successful production of pellagra in strong, healthy white males by a faulty diet. At the National Association meeting, he could not mention research which was still underway and still under a cloak of secrecy, yet when Goldberger was in the news again in less than two weeks, it seemed, in retrospect, as if he had been hiding something. Some who had praised him at the Columbia meeting joined a new chorus which berated him roundly.

The research was carried out at Rankin Prison Farm, eight miles east of Jackson, Mississippi. That state, harder hit by pellagra than any other in the South, was anxious to cooperate in any plan that seemed to offer a solution to the pellagra riddle. In 1914 there had been 1,192 deaths from pellagra in Mississippi, and in 1915 this figure rose to a high of 1,531.[64] Governor Earl Brewer was most concerned. Impressed by Goldberger's work at the orphanages, he authorized the new pellagra experiment, and Galloway, secretary of the Mississippi State Board of Health, arranged the details. It was Galloway, in fact, who persuaded the governor to make the test possible. Goldberger called him "our good angel."[65] The governor promised a pardon to any twelve men in the prison farm who volunteered to participate.

The plan was to induce pellagra in white adult males, the one group in the population that statistics had shown was the least likely to contract the disease. Goldberger reasoned that if a good diet prevented pellagra, a bad one ought to induce it. He would feed prisoners a restricted, mainly cereal diet not unlike that which thousands of people in the South sat down to every day. Although there was pellagra in abundance in Mississippi, there had never been a case on the 3,200 acre Rankin Farm. The seventy to eighty convicts regularly quartered there were in good health.

The convict camp was at the center of the farm. Inside a stockade, surrounded by a board fence, were four buildings: the "cage" where the prisoners slept, the old hospital, the dining hall, and the church. The prisoners who volunteered for Goldberger's test moved to the "new hospital," a small one-story cottage of recent construction located just outside the stockade. Compared to the "cage," it was very clean. The new hospital was thoroughly overhauled before the prisoners moved in. It was carefully screened and repaired so that the flies, mosquitoes, fleas, and bedbugs, which had such ready access to the other buildings at Rankin Prison Farm, would be kept out of this one building.[66]

The "pellagra squad," as the dozen volunteers were called, was organized early in February 1915. They were moved at once to the new hospital and placed under a special day-and-night guard. In April, one attempted to escape and was replaced by another volunteer. In July, one had to drop out because of another illness, leaving eleven to complete the test. The squad members included six who were serving life terms for murder, one a life term for criminal assault, and the others lesser terms for manslaughter, bigamy, and embezzlement. The two embezzlers were the most interesting of the group. They were wealthy brothers, E. S. and Woodson Atkinson of Summit, Mississippi, who had served half of their seven-year terms. Ranked among the wealthiest and most influential citizens of their county, these one-time bank officers had been convicted of embezzlement after their bank crashed. It may have been a gambling spirit that prompted them to be the first to volunteer.[67]

The pellagra squad did the same work as other prisoners on the farm. They whitewashed fences and buildings, cut weeds and grass, baled hay, and sawed lumber. They rested two-and-a-half days a week. As the experiment progressed and the men grew weaker, they rested more and more, and, during the final week, they did no work at all. To be certain they had no contact with pellagra they were strictly segregated. As an added precaution, they bathed regularly, wore clean clothes, and scrubbed all the furniture in the dormitory once a week.[68]

The diet of the squad differed sharply from that of the prisoners who served as controls for the experiment. For the first ten weeks, everyone at the farm, pellagra squad and all, ate the same food—the regular diet of the camp, which was restricted enough, consisting as it did largely of biscuit, cornbread, cured pork, and syrup. It did contain, however, some fresh beef, pork, and kid, beans and peas, and eggs occasionally. During the summer months, the diet was more varied with a marked increase in the use of milk and fresh vegetables, particularly greens. The approximate average composition of the regular diet of the convicts was 3,500 to 4,000 calories a day, of which 10 to 11 percent was derived from protein.

On April 19, the pellagra squad began the new diet, one that was mostly carbohydrates. It provided the men with from

2,500 to 3,500 calories a day, but only 6 percent of these came from protein, and this protein was from cereal sources. For breakfast, the men were served biscuits, mush, rice, gravy, syrup, coffee, and sugar; for dinner, corn bread, collards, sweet potatoes, grits, and syrup; for supper, biscuits, mush, grits, gravy, syrup, coffee, and sugar. For variety, the breakfast rice and the supper grits were sometimes switched. Until late July buttermilk was used in making wheat biscuits; then this was eliminated. Only once was there any change. In late June, Dr. George A. Wheeler, the PHS officer whom Goldberger left in charge of the prison experiment, gave in to growing complaints of the volunteers and served a little meat. There were three pounds of beefsteak for one meal; each man got about four ounces.[69]

The experiment was conducted under increasingly trying conditions. At first the men treated the whole experiment as a lark; it all seemed so easy. Within two weeks, however, there was a complaint. One of the Atkinson brothers felt weak and dizzy. Six days later, his brother had pains in his stomach. By the third week of June, all the prisoners were complaining in one way or another. They lost weight and suffered from pains in their backs and sides or cramps in their legs. Some had sore mouths and tongues. A few developed the increased knee jerk typical of what the medical profession had come to call "pellagra sine pellagra," this is, pellagra without visible skin manifestations. One man said he was just "no 'count'" and was "about played out." Another said he was weak and nervous. As dramatic as the physical changes were, the mental changes were even more startling. One of the volunteers, a man of great physical strength with an exceptionally jovial disposition, boasted in late May of his strength and good health. Within the week, however, he announced he was going to die and that he could not possibly survive the test. He became very quiet, refusing even to speak to the other volunteers and was so moody that other members of the pellagra squad were afraid of him. The first skin lesions did not appear on any of the volunteers until September 12, or about the end of the fifth month of the experiment. By the end of that month, several others also had a suspicious looking rash.

It first appeared on the scrotum, and later on the hands of two of the men and on the back of the neck of another. Its appearance intensified the growing uneasiness of the volunteers. When the rash was first spotted on the ring finger of one of the men, he was extremely nervous and insisted that it was caused by cylinder grease which he had got on his hand while baling hay.[70] The appearance of the rash, while upsetting to the volunteers, brought unmitigated joy to Goldberger and to Wheeler. It was late appearing, and, as the mandatory six-months deadline for the end of the experiment approached, Wheeler was afraid that the whole thing would have to be considered a failure. Although the volunteers had shown quite early in the experiment the symptoms of pellagra sine pellagra, no definite diagnosis of pellagra could be made without the characteristic skin rash, and for a time, it seemed as if this would not appear. The diagnosis of pellagra in six of the eleven men was confirmed by four experienced physicians.[71]

"I do not yet realize that we have really and truly produced pellagra in great big, vigorous men by just feeding them properly or rather 'improperly,'" the happy Goldberger wrote his wife. "This is way beyond anything I had anticipated. The most I had hoped for; the most I prayed for was two cases. We have five! Isn't that enough to daze one and to make one doubtful of one's senses!"[72]

Part of the agreement with the volunteers was that after they received their pardons they might return to the prison farm for a proper diet so that they could regain their health. Not one of the volunteers took advantage of this offer. The official reports said that they "passed from observation." Goldberger expressed it more accurately when he said that they "all went off like a lot of scared rabbits."[73]

The scene in the governor's office when the prisoners received their pardons was a dramatic one. A Baptist minister was there to offer prayer for their recovery and for their return to useful life. The men arrived at the Capitol in their prison stripes. Tears rolled down their cheeks as they stepped up to receive their pardons. At the end of the ceremony, pardons in hand, they marched out to receive the customary suit of clothes and five dollars. Later, some of them told what the experiment had been like. "I have been through a thousand hells," one man put it, adding that often he would have welcomed a bullet.[74]

Two men wrote the governor before the experiment was over, begging to be released from the pellagra squad. They said they preferred a lifetime of hard labor to living through another week of this "hellish experiment." Efforts had been made to keep the experiment secret until it was over and results could be announced. Governor Brewer feared that if relatives of the prisoners knew what was taking place, they would institute habeas corpus proceedings to get the men released from the squad. But word of the activities at the Rankin Prison Farm leaked out anyway, and the governor was bitterly assailed for permitting the test. He was also accused of staging it as an excuse to grant pardons to the Atkinson brothers. Goldberger, however, had nothing but praise for the governor. He said science and humanity were forever in his debt.[75]

The prison experiment contained all the elements of sensational news, and Mississippi newspapers made the most of it with big headlines and front-page stories. The national press took due notice of it as well. The prominence given the story was enough to rankle those members of the medical profession who objected to flamboyant announcements of medical progress, especially if the ideas so heralded did not happen to coincide with their own. Goldberger had no such qualms. After the proof offered in the prison experiment, he considered as "hopeless" anybody who still doubted that pellagra was essentially of dietary origin. He was convinced that with those people, time alone could deal adequately.[76] It did take quite a long time to deal with these "hopeless" ones, whose number appeared to be legion. The storm was about to burst.

4

Praise and
Protest

GOLDBERGER HAD A brief moment of glory in Jackson when results of the prison experiment were announced. The *Jackson Daily News* headlined the story "DISEASE ROBBED OF TERRORS" and placed Goldberger in the ranks of the South's medical heroes, alongside Reed and Carroll who had sacrificed their lives in yellow-fever research. The Jackson Rotary Club made him an honorary member, and, according to press dispatches, the doctor was showered with congratulatory telegrams from all parts of the United States, chiefly from members of the medical profession. Goldberger bore his honors well. The *Daily News* described him as "exceedingly modest." For two days he dodged congratulations, refused to talk about the tests, and would not grant interviews. His next assignment, the press observed, would probably be an even more baffling problem, maybe even cancer.[1]

It was cause for comment that Goldberger's "wonderful discovery" brought him international renown but no financial reward. As a Public Health Service employee, his salary remained exactly the same. Goldberger was, as a matter of fact, at that very moment nursing his disappointment at not being selected as director of the Hygienic Laboratory. He had applied for the post in August, while the prison experiment was still underway, and learned in late October that it had gone to someone else. "Of course, I wanted it and perhaps I'm disappointed but I do really feel that the disappointment is barely skin deep," he wrote home. "There is one thing I can say that I have produced pellagra by diet! I don't care who is director."[2]

Praise for success of the prison experiment helped soothe his wounded vanity, but he did not have long to savor compliments. Repercussions came almost immediately. These ranged from picayune criticisms by laymen, who thought that, if more "noble lives" than those of prisoners had been used for the experiment, results would have been more heroic, to those of medical men who objected to so much publicity for a test conducted in secret.[3]

It was at the meeting of the Southern Medical Association in Dallas, Texas, just one week after the dramatic announcement of the success of the prison experiment, that protests against Goldberger, his work, and his theory reached a crescendo. The pellagra symposium held at the meeting did not accept diet as a positive cure. Rather, one speaker after another rejected the newly minted diet theory in favor of well-worn old favorites. Pellagra was blamed variously on corn bread, Italian immigrants, amoebas, cane sugar, and infection. Only a few of those attending the session came to Goldberger's defense.[4]

The meeting was more than a forum for physicians to speak up once more in favor of their own pet theories. It was a sounding board for a vitriolic attack on Goldberger, who was not present. The report on his work was read by Dr. Allan W. Freeman of the Public Health Service, a report which indicated that the diet used to cause pellagra was almost identical to that of every person of small means in the South. Freeman defended his fellow health officer's views, but added that it was "perhaps unfortunate" that Goldberger had announced his findings so soon.[5]

Loudest in his denunciation of the prison project was Hayne,

who just three weeks before had "bleated very gently" and withdrawn his own paper at the meeting of the National Association
for the Study of Pellagra. Hayne did not bleat gently at the
SMA meeting. He stormed. He was upset by accounts of the
prison experiment, which he had read on the train en route
to Dallas. He objected strenuously to opinions on pellagra being
published in the lay press, for, he said, it was so hard to get
out of the minds of people ideas they had picked up by reading
the newspapers. He predicted that the theory of pellagra's being
caused by diet alone would be exploded just like the one that
malaria was caused by bad water. Almost as loud was Dr. John
Jelks of Memphis, the staunch champion of the amebic theory
of pellagra, who exclaimed "Eureka!" when he saw the great
headlines in the *Memphis Commercial Appeal*. He thought such
publicity constituted a double standard of ethics; it represented
an effort to make doctors choke down knowledge which would
have been more acceptable in an age of superstition. Another
Memphis doctor, Louis Leroy, drew applause when he described as "pernicious" the newspaper publicity that told people
there was no danger of pellagra except from poor food and
cooking. Another doctor from Arkansas said he would not insult
the doctors' intelligence by trying to pretend that pellagra was
anything other than infectious. One might as well try to prove
that wet weather was the cause of the boll weevil as to try
to prove that pellagra was due to an unbalanced diet.

There were one or two doctors at the meeting who defended
Goldberger's work. Most outspoken of these was Dr. Charles
W. Garrison, state health officer of Arkansas, who challenged
the statement that publication of an adequate diet was injurious
either to the people or the profession. In his state where a campaign "Let Arkansas Feed Herself" was underway, pellagra was
being used to prod the movement alone. Since every doctor at
the Dallas meeting indicated an adequate diet was fundamental
to treatment of the disease, even if they disagreed most violently
that it was the only treatment, Garrison thought it worthwhile

.

to let people know they were eating an unbalanced diet and that, if possible, they should keep a cow.[6]

The *Jackson Daily News,* which took a sort of proprietary interest in Goldberger's work, was incensed about criticism of Mississippi's newest hero. The jealousy existing among comic opera soubrettes was "mild and harmless indeed when compared to the pea-green envy frequently shown among members of the medical profession," the paper observed editorially. Why should Goldberger have made his prison experiments public through medical journals that nobody but doctors would read? The "pill-passers" who criticized Goldberger's work were simply jealous. "An honest, sincere practitioner ought to be glad to accept the Goldberger theory at face value, and put it immediately into practice, since it is the only rational treatment that has yet been offered for the dread disease that is killing thousands of people in the South each year. Mean and narrow-minded indeed must be the medico who would deliberately seek to destroy the hope that has been given birth in the minds of many sufferers within the past few days."[7]

The Dallas meeting was a study in miniature of what Goldberger once described as the two-centuries old "impressionistic school" of research—one in which the researcher, after turning in his chair and looking at a long distance out the window, announced solemnly his mature impression of scientific facts. During all that time no one had tried the curative effect of diet alone. Rather, as strong believers in the possibility of mining pure scientific gold, members of this school believed the problem to be a matter for the brain rather than for the hand. They deemed the intricate processes of refinement unnecessary. Goldberger thought these processes to be essential, even though simple. His own dictum in analyzing results was that a promising result once might be an accident; twice it might be a coincidence; but a promising result three times was proof positive.[8]

Bolstered by evidence he considered proof positive, Goldberger was seemingly impervious to criticism heaped on his head at

Dallas. An associate of Goldberger's in the PHS, Dr. R. C. Williams, has observed that it was "characteristic of [him] to be perfectly oblivious to personal interest when engaged in his official duties, and like a faithful soldier he received his wounds with philosophy and with no abatement of zeal."[9]

A few days after the Dallas meeting, en route to a meeting of health officers in Little Rock, he said he expected to be kept busy dodging verbal brickbats, but that he looked forward to the onslaught with "entire calm and peace." At Little Rock, however, he was pleasantly surprised. Few, if any, brickbats were thrown. Instead he encountered one man who said that he had "swallowed Dr. Goldberger whole," and another who claimed that his only objection to the "Goldberger treatment" was that his patients had seen so much about diet in the newspapers that they refused to take medicine. " 'Diet' has taken root; it will grow; it will spread abroad," Goldberger wrote home. Opposition to it would only help spread the good news. Although he appeared oblivious to criticism, privately he was annoyed and angry. He called those who disagreed with him "blind, selfish, jealous, prejudiced asses."[10]

The outburst against Goldberger broke out anew at the meeting of the Tri-State Medical Association in Memphis that same month. It was, as the *Jackson Daily News* again commented editorially, a "hammer-on-the-anvil chorus" against him, one which it was difficult for the layman to understand. The *Daily News* suggested that perhaps Goldberger's theory was too simple, his advice too easy to follow. A pellagra sufferer could cure himself. Specifically, doctors at this meeting objected to Goldberger's calling in so few physicians to witness the prison experiment. They claimed that those who were called to examine the pellagra squad might have been biased in their views. They also objected to the idea that was implicit in the whole dietary theory: that the South was starving its people. This struck a tender cord. There were loud protests that Southerners were living better than ever, yet they had more pellagra. And, as if to underscore this point, there was an occasional reference to the well-to-do, those with plenty of money to buy food, who sometimes suffered from the disease. Yet the association of pellagra with the South's poverty was not to be denied. Even those who objected most strenuously to Goldberger and his theory admitted it. An Arkansas doctor observed that the best preventive of pellagra was $200 in the bank. Another from Tennessee said that the whole diet theory was impossible because pellagrins were so poor. One might as well tell a pauper to take a "jaunt on the ocean's wave and to inhale the fragrant breezes of faraway Araby" as to tell him to drink milk and eat tenderloin beef. He implied that medicine was cheaper and more satisfactory than good food.[11]

The most bitter attack on Goldberger was made by Dr. MacNeal of the Thompson–McFadden Commission who wrote a two-and-a-half page diatribe about the prison experiment for *JAMA*. He objected particularly to the fact that Goldberger had said nothing about his "alleged important discovery" at the recent meeting of the National Association for the Study of Pellagra. He was also angry because such recognized authorities as Dr. Lavinder, president of the NASP, and Dr. Siler, vice president of the same group, were not invited to see "such alleged important cases."

Goldberger's response to MacNeal's charge was short, cool, and precise and might have been interpreted as weak by those unfamiliar with his style. It would have been "premature" to have mentioned the prison experiment at the South Carolina meeting, Goldberger said, since the dermatitis developed gradually and was not recognized as significant until after the date of the meeting. Lavinder and Siler had not been called in simply because the experiment had to be terminated abruptly: the six months allocated for it had expired.[12]

Criticism of Goldberger's work appeared in at least two books the year after the prison experiment. William H. Deaderick and L. D. Thompson in their *Endemic Diseases of the Southern*

States agreed basically with Goldberger's recommendations on diet, but said the prison experiment would have been more convincing had it been carried out in a pellagra-free territory.[13] A much stronger criticism came from Dr. E. M. Perdue of Kansas City, Missouri, who called the prison experiment "silly" and predicted that the sacrifice of a few thousand more lives would "perhaps repay these officials for their attempt to block the way of therapeutic progress."[14] Perdue had his own idea about the cause of pellagra, one he had picked up from two Italian scientists and adapted for the American scene. He thought it was caused by drinking "soft" or "freestone" water common to clay soil districts. Perdue's book was an extensive elaboration of an idea he had advanced in a letter to Governor Brewer shortly after the prison experiment results were announced. Likening Goldberger's project to medieval torture, he said it demanded the "execration and scathing denunciation of all reasonable men." Governor Brewer, a reasonable man, advised Perdue not to criticize other people's work unless he could do better himself. "Show me," he said. Produce pellagra through the use of freestone water, and the governor would then be convinced.[15]

While most of the attacks on Goldberger came from those who disagreed with his theories, there was at least one from a man of like persuasion who was angry because he had not received credit and publicity. This was Carl Voegtlin of the government's Pellagra Hospital in Spartanburg, who claimed to have been the first to suggest that pellagra was a dietary deficiency disease. The entire program of the hospital at Spartanburg, much of which he had worked out, was based on a test of deficiencies of a mainly vegetable diet. Voegtlin was convinced that the etiology of pellagra was far from being established, that much more work had to be done, and that if all Goldberger's recommendations must be accepted, the hospital might just as well be closed.[16]

Voegtlin's attitude toward Goldberger may well have been

based on jealousy, but the reticence of other doctors to accept his ideas is not so easily explained. They resented an "outsider's" coming in and finding so much fault with the South's diet, but, more important, they were not ready to accept a new concept of medicine, one that seemed to fly in the face of all they had learned about the nature of disease. They had hardly become accustomed to the "new knowledge" that diseases were caused by bacteria when Goldberger discarded this idea in the case of pellagra for one that seemed altogether improbable.

Until about 1905, public health work in the Southeast was based on the idea that disease was caused by filth. The decomposition of animal and vegetable matter gave rise to poisonous gases or germs, which fell on people or were breathed in by them causing epidemic diseases. Health authorities in those years concerned themselves with cleaning up the environment, looking for possible sources of disease in the public dump, in piles of decaying leaves, or in poorly designed cesspools. About the turn of the century, and certainly by 1905, public health officials of the South, reflecting new advances in medicine, embraced the bacteriological concept of disease.[17] Successful campaigns against yellow fever gave this concept deservedly high esteem. It seemed foolish to abandon an approach which they had just discovered worked so well.

New ideas do not go unchallenged. Not even Robert Koch's discovery of the tubercle bacillus in 1882 was readily accepted. He himself predicted it would take two generations for medical men to accept the relationship between the great white plague and the tubercle bacillus. Anybody with a trained eye and a microscope could see it, but there were many who continued to blame tuberculosis on heredity. The great "Philadelphia debate" of 1883 on the cause of tuberculosis might be compared to the great Southern debate of 1915 and later on the cause of pellagra. At least Koch and his defenders could support their arguments by something that could be seen. Goldberger could only talk about something mysteriously missing. Physicians had finally become used to Koch's ideas, to thinking about positive causes of diseases. It took an entirely different mental framework to think of disease in terms of a lack.[18]

When Goldberger began work on pellagra, the science of nutrition was in its infancy. In the late eighteenth century, Lavoisier had found that man was a machine capable of using the energy of carbohydrates and fats in food for his own activities. For a hundred years, interest in nutrition centered on this aspect. The only new idea in a century was that some protein was essential for growth and existence and that certain mineral and other inorganic elements were also necessary. By the end of the century, men had learned to measure the energy or calories in proteins, fats, and carbohydrates. Give a man enough calories for his needs, and his diet was adequate. In 1897, Professor W. O. Atwater of Maine, who devised the technique of measuring calories, deprecated the use of green vegetables since they contained only small amounts of protein and provided little energy. He maintained that vegetables were necessary only to render the diet palatable and supply bulk and mineral salts.

Work in animal nutrition at the University of Wisconsin during the early years of the twentieth century, as well as studies at Yale University, revealed that the quality of proteins differs. Only then was attention turned to the qualitative aspects of nutrition. It was not until 1912 that Professor Elmer V. McCollum at Wisconsin's Agricultural Experiment Station discovered the first vitamin, a fat-soluble substance he named "A" for lack of a better term, something so essential in the diet that, without it, rats did not grow well, could not raise young, and suffered from xerophthalmia.

In 1915 when the attack on Goldberger was at its height, most medical men did not know much chemistry. Work in nutrition was being done by chemists, not physicians. Fascinated with improved microscopes and new techniques of staining, physicians could not think of metabolic processes in terms of chemical systems. As McCollum pointed out, "they did not comprehend the idea that deficiency of some specific chemical substance could cause derangement of physiological processes and result in pathological states."[19] It was not until after 1915 that new criteria were adopted to assess the quality in human and animal foods. The discovery of vitamins, the demonstration of specific kinds of deficiencies in individual natural foods, and the proven effectiveness of milk, egg yolk, and leafy vegetables as supplements to a diet of purified nutrients led to important advances. Goldberger's work in pellagra would eventually help physicians accept work the chemists were doing.

Southern physicians who denied the validity of Goldberger's work were not the only ones who could not think of disease as being caused by a lack of something. In 1917, McCollum, who by then had moved to Johns Hopkins University in Baltimore, found that many highly trained medical men, biologists, and pathologists were not willing to accept the new viewpoints that experimental work in nutrition had brought to light. He attributed it to lethargy. For half a century, erroneous beliefs in grossly oversimplified concepts of diet had hardly been disturbed. Farmers admired experimentalists in animal feeding, but only a few people believed this work to be of importance in solving problems of human nutrition.[20]

There was historical precedent, too, for not accepting Goldberger's findings on pellagra. It was forty-eight years after James Lind published *A Treatise on Scurvy* in 1753, which showed that two oranges and a lemon a day would cure this scourge of the sea, before the British Royal Navy began regular use of lemon or lime juice on long voyages. More recently, Eijkman and Grinjns's demonstration that whole grain rice would prevent beriberi was hotly debated from the first announcement of their findings in 1896 to 1912. During those sixteen years, more than six hundred writers expressed skepticism and offered other theories.[21]

Goldberger had no plan for communicating his ideas to the public, and he said as much in an interview with the press when results of the prison experiment were announced: "It is hardly part of my duty to offer any advice or suggestions along this line. In fact, I have not matured any plans in my own mind."[22] Naively, perhaps, he believed that having pointed the way, physicians and state health departments would follow his lead.

This was before the great uproar. Within a couple of months he had concluded that the only way to get his gospel of diet accepted was to skip over physicians and convince intelligent laymen he was right. He explained his ideas to Dr. Charles T. Nesbitt, public health officer of Wilmington, North Carolina, during a visit to that city in January 1916.

Nesbitt quizzed Goldberger about why he permitted and even sought lay publicity. Goldberger's reasons were simple. He believed it to be the quickest way to change medical opinion. Newspapers and magazines reached thinking men and women who then put pressure on the medical profession. When a doctor found a layman outstripping him in knowledge he was generally supposed to possess, he was under the painful necessity of catching up and getting ahead. Goldberger hoped to break the vicious circle of an "unthinking public and a half-educated commercialized medical profession" acting and reacting on each other. The wedge he wanted to use was that of the thinking citizen.[23]

Nesbitt did not have to be won over by a thinking citizen. He was impressed with Goldberger the man, and found him to be one of the most interesting people he had ever met. Nesbitt was, in fact, surprised at the new opinion he formed of Goldberger's work after meeting the man in person. The carefully written reports issued by the Public Health Service had not given him the correct impression of work the man had done, and he found the popular idea of his work created in the public press to be very misleading. "The real essentials of his work have been missed," he wrote a friend. "Everybody who has written about it had injected a little damn foolishness into it just enough to render turbid its really crystalline simplicity." In Nesbitt's opinion, Goldberger was of the "high-type class of scientific investigators."[24]

Nesbitt was not the only one whom Goldberger won over in Wilmington. He addressed a meeting of thirty or forty physicians from the area who were of widely varying opinions before the lecture. There was but one who raised objections afterward, and this one had the "legs gently pulled from under him. . . . Dr. Goldberger made himself so clear that the others simply laughed at the doubting Thomas." Within two months after Goldberger's visit, Dr. Edward J. Wood, whom Goldberger described as "the bed bug man," was holding a clinic in the basement of the court house for the instruction of pellagra patients and treatment of cases according to the Goldberger method. There was not a doctor in town who had not accepted the diet idea.[25]

The visit to Wilmington provided a brief haven in the midst of a storm. Another respite came a few months later when Goldberger received support from an unexpected quarter—the Thompson–McFadden Commission. Captain Edward B. Vedder of the Army Medical Corps, working for the commission, stated the case for diet. He conducted a month's investigation in the Spartanburg area in the summer of 1914 and immediately wrote his report, but it was not published until two years later. He saw a striking resemblance between pellagra and beriberi, a disease known to be caused by poor diet. Like beriberi, pellagra was a disease of the poor, with an extraordinary frequency in hospitals for the insane. He suggested the reason the disease reappeared each spring was that its victims had a deficient diet all winter, and that it disappeared in the fall because the summer's fare was so much better. This was comparable to Goldberger's view that pellagra was a "spring crop." Unlike the commission which hired him, Vedder could find no relationship between the location of the house in which one lived and the incidence of pellagra. Rather, he said, location of a man's house was but an indication of his economic status. It was natural that poor people would live in one section of a community and the well-to-do in another. Thus pellagra, being a disease of the poor, would appear in clumps wherever the poor were segregated from the rest of the community.

Vedder found fault with the inexact terms that the commission used in its dietary survey. It was not accurate enough, he maintained, to ask if a person used a certain food "daily, habitually, rarely, or never" as the commission had done. He suggested the possibility that some deficiency in wheat flour was responsible for pellagra, since this flour composed such a large part of the diet of the Southern poor. He said the dietary theory explained why women were so much more susceptible to pellagra than men. Women were most likely to become pellagrins in the child-bearing years between twenty and forty. A diet sufficient for their needs in ordinary circumstances could not preserve their health under the additional stress of pregnancy. And, as Vedder observed, there was no "race suicide" in the South. A family of five to eight children was quite usual.[26]

In comparing pellagra to beriberi, Vedder spoke as an authority. For three years before he made the Spartanburg study, he had worked in the Philippine Islands as a member of the army board for the study of tropical diseases, and in 1913 had won the Cartwright Prize of Columbia University for his book *Beriberi*. He had observed hundreds of polyneuritis cases and had seen victims at the point of death recover when given an extract of rice polishings. Working with a young chemist, R. R. Williams, Vedder tried without success to isolate the factor responsible for the cures. He found the same substance in yeast that he found in rice and puzzled over what to call it. Because he thought it unreasonable to give the substance a different name for each food stuff in which it happened to be a constituent, he referred to it as a vitamin, the term coined by Funk. At the University of Wisconsin, McCollum labeled it vitamin B, the second accessory food factor to be discovered.[27]

Vedder knew that beriberi could be cured by the simple expedient of eating whole grain rather than polished rice, but he recognized the difficulties of educating people to eat what was good for them rather than what they liked. A paragraph in his book pointed up the problems involved, and he predicted that such a dietary education program would cause great difficulties even in the United States.

> To me it appears that any such educational campaign is doomed to failure because of the magnitude of the undertaking, and because those who propose it fail to take into consideration the inertia and disinclination of oriental peoples to change their habits. Some conception of the magnitude of the undertaking may be obtained if we imagine a similar condition in the United States or Europe. Let us suppose, for instance, that some serious disease such as cancer were caused by eating white bread and that it could be entirely prevented by eating whole wheat bread. How long would it take us by a campaign of education to change the habits of the entire people and induce them all to eat whole grain wheat bread? Europeans and Americans are intelligent and not constitutionally opposed to a change of custom, yet it must be admitted it would require years to effect such a change, probably at least a decade. All intelligent people know that typhoid is a disease contracted directly from an antecedent case of the same disease, yet whole cities still continue to use diluted sewage for their drinking supply, from streams which everyone knows are grossly contaminated. To effect such a radical change in the staple food of an oriental people by education alone would require a long time, if indeed it could be accomplished at all. And in the meantime they would still suffer from beriberi, a disease that is clearly preventable.[28]

Vedder suggested the problem of beriberi might be solved by a prohibitively high tax on polished rice.

If Goldberger read Vedder's book, he knew a hard job lay ahead of him. Apparently it was not enough to show doctors that good diet alone would cure pellagra, and the process of educating the public would surely be long and tedious. Vedder thought it would take a decade. It was to take much longer than that.

Nevertheless, the work began. Most of the state health departments in the South were cooperative, in spite of an occasional blast from one of them. Even Hayne of South Carolina, despite misgivings about Goldberger's methods, included in his annual report for 1915 the suggestion that a propaganda campaign be launched in the state to educate the people to the necessity of eating a more varied diet. In Louisiana a lumber company at Bogalusa set up a hospital to treat pellagra patients at the company's expense and asked for Goldberger's help. Louisiana parishes considered for a time the feasibility of setting up camps near pellagrous communities to provide relief. Florida also began work through its board of health to eradicate the disease, and Mississippi laid elaborate plans for educating the public on proper diet. On the heels of the announcement of the successful prison experiment, the *Jackson Daily News* printed Goldberger's complete pellagra remedy from the advice to eat more meat and fewer carbohydrates to the necessity of improving economic conditions.[29]

It was imperative that Mississippi do something to control pellagra. The year 1915 saw the number of cases climb to 15,831, about 10 percent of whom died. This was a ratio of almost 80 cases per 100,000 people. Hospitals refused patients with the disease, and in many counties local resources were severely taxed to care for the ill.[30] The state health board worked hard to reduce the toll. It left thousands of bulletins at country stores throughout the state telling people in the simplest language what they should eat. It also asked the legislature for help. The board itself felt helpless to do anything with such an enormous problem without an appropriation for this specific purpose. The funds with which it had to work were not enough. When the legislature convened in early December 1915, there was on every desk a copy of a carefully prepared study in which the board stated the need and outlined a plan.

The Mississippi plan was based on total acceptance of the dietary theory. If pellagra were caused by a one-sided diet, it should not be too difficult to cure. If the cost of milk, fresh lean meat, and eggs made them prohibitive, then Mississippians could eat beans. Farmers should be urged to keep cows and chickens, raise meat, and plant beans; teachers should be required to tell pupils what caused pellagra; and everyone should be urged to eat beans, if they could not do better, especially in the late winter and spring months. The death rate from pellagra jumped by more than 47 percent in 1914. Health authorities feared it would continue to rise until the state and the counties educated people on the cause of the disease and made some provision for treating those already ill. Dependence on the public press alone was not enough.

The health board appealed for support of its educational program for business as well as for humanitarian reasons: pellagra was expensive in Mississippi. Estimated cost of the disease in the state in 1914 was conservatively put at $2,280,111. This included time lost from work, cost of medicine and funerals, and loss in human life, valued at $1,500 each. If life were considered of no value, the cost was still $478,611 for one year. To save this much money and to prevent suffering and death, the health board asked for an appropriation of $30,000 for pellagra work. In the same breath, the department admitted that the chance of getting this much money was slim.

Specifically, the health board wanted enough money to hire eight physicians as field men to make house-to-house calls in their territories, give instruction on what constituted an adequate diet, and distribute literature. The need for more printed literature was urgent. Calls came every day for it, not only from people in Mississippi but from those in other states as well. If the state assumed the education job, counties could assume responsibility for treatment. County camps for treatment of pellagra were suggested. These were to be constructed cheaply with just enough precaution to prevent spread of typhoid, malaria, and other diseases which could be even more fatal than pellagra.[31] The health board did get authorization for county pellagra hospitals. A bill giving counties authority to erect these, financed through issuance of bonds, was passed in April 1916.[32]

That the task of educating the public was difficult Goldberger knew only too well. He could not convince even some associates in the Public Health Service that diet was the answer. He was greatly disturbed about a report appearing in an Atlanta newspaper in September 1918 that a Public Health Service physician had accidentally discovered a quick cure for pellagra, one that worked in three weeks instead of the "year and a half required by other methods." Goldberger wrote Surgeon General Blue protesting that such stories interfered with proper education of the public, a matter of great importance in public health.[33] He was disturbed, too, that advertisements for "pellagra cures" continued to appear regularly in the press. Medicine would only alleviate painful symptoms; it would not cure the disease. The sooner this is realized the sooner the quacks, both within and without the profession, will be put out of business, he wrote in *Public Health Reports:* "The money that is now being wasted on useless and quack medicines is well-nigh sufficient to procure for the poor, deluded sufferers the food from the lack of which they are suffering."[34]

The educational campaign paid good dividends in Mississippi, where the incidence of pellagra in 1916 was cut to half what it had been the year before. This drop was attributed to "very different financial and food conditions" in the state that year as well as to wide publicity given the need for a good diet.[35] Any decrease was welcome. No accurate statistics were available on the number of cases in the South as a whole; only in Mississippi were relatively complete records kept. The lowest estimate of pellagra cases in the South in 1915 was about 75,000, with approximately 7,500 deaths. The highest estimate was 0.5 percent of the South's entire population of 32.5 million, or 165,000 pellagrins.[36] In many areas only tuberculosis and pneumonia outranked it as a cause of death.

Goldberger himself believed the fatality rate was not more than 5 percent. Thus, he considered pellagra to be more important as a cause of sickness which lowered physical efficiency than as a cause of death, important as this might be. He said there were probably 70,000 definite cases of pellagra in the six-state area of Mississippi, Alabama, South Carolina, North Carolina, Tennessee, and Texas in 1916. Assuming that there were at least half that many more in the remaining seven Southern states, he fixed the number of cases for that year at upward of 100,000.[37]

As the months passed, Goldberger refined his thinking on pellagra. He did not know the specific missing quantity in a pellagrin's diet, just as Vedder did not know specifically what the body required to prevent beriberi. In time he hoped to find the missing nutrient. In time he also hoped to prove statistically what he already believed to be true—that pellagra and economics were intimately related. Meanwhile, he thought his educational campaign would receive a boost if he could spike the arguments of his opposition, the infectionists. The only way to do this was to prove definitely, scientifically, that they were wrong.

He designed an experiment, an unpleasant one, which he thought would quiet the opposition. It consisted of a series of "filth parties" in which one final effort would be made to transmit disease from a pellagrin to another living creature. This time, however, neither monkeys, baboons, guinea pigs nor rabbits were the experimental animals. There was always the possibility that these animals were immune. Man, however, was definitely not immune. In this final test, Goldberger, fourteen of his associates, and his wife took the place of laboratory animals.

On seven different occasions from late April to the end of June 1916, Goldberger tried to contract pellagra himself or give it to one of his associates. He used all the time-honored ways of experimentally transmitting a disease, employing every known method of infection: blood, nasal secretions, epidermal scales from skin lesions, urine, and feces. He took part in all seven experiments, Mrs. Goldberger in one.

The first experiment was conducted at the Pellagra Hospital in Spartanburg where blood was drawn from the elbow of a pellagrin and injected into Goldberger's left shoulder muscle and that of his associate from the prison experiment, George Wheeler. Both reported some stiffness in the shoulder, but nothing more. Three days later at the State Hospital for the Insane in Columbia, South Carolina, Goldberger took some scales and urine from two pellagra patients and feces from a third, worked them into a wheat flour pill, and swallowed it. He participated in this test alone. Except for diarrhea which lasted about a week, he suffered no ill effects.[38]

By May 7, he was ready for the third experiment, the one in which Mrs. Goldberger took part. She received an injection of blood only. The other five participants, received similar injections and also swallowed "pills" like those Goldberger had first tested on himself. Later one of the volunteers noticed an enlarged and somewhat tender lymph gland near where the blood was injected. That was the only ill effect. The fourth experiment was noted in the Medical Officers Journal of the Hygienic Laboratory:

> June 7, 1916—In order to contribute data for the solution of the problem of the infectious or non-infectious nature of Pellagra the following officers of the service submitted to a feeding experiment conducted by Surgeon Joseph Goldberger, in charge of Pellagra Investigations:
>
> Assistant Surgeon General R. H. Creel
> Surgeon Joseph Goldberger
> Surgeon G. W. McCoy
> Surgeon A. M. Stimson
> Surgeon E. A. Sweet
> Passed Assistant Surgeon W. F. Draper
> George W. McCoy
> Director
>

McCoy signed twice, once as a participant, once as director of the laboratory.[39]

Similar experiments were carried out three times more in Washington, New Orleans, and Spartanburg. Several volunteers had diarrhea for a week or more, one felt somewhat nauseated, and two had mild dyspepsia. But there was never any sign of pellagra, and no volunteer suffered any permanent ill effects. Considering the "relatively enormous quantities of filth taken" Goldberger noted, "the reactions experienced were surprisingly light."[40]

"We had our final 'filth party' . . . this noon," Goldberger wrote in late June from Spartanburg where he and two associates had gathered for the last test. "If anyone ever got pellagra that way, we three should certainly have it good and hard! We just feasted on filth. It's the last time. Never again!"[41]

Mrs. Goldberger testified years later that it took no courage to take part in these experiments. Rather, it was an act of faith. Goldberger found his faulty diet theory "materially strengthened" by these new tests.[42]

To avoid violent repercussions from premature publicity, no announcement was made of these experiments until November 1916, when Goldberger read his paper before the meeting of the Southern Medical Association in Atlanta. His was but one of four papers in a symposium on pellagra, but when the meeting was opened for discussion, his might have been the only one presented. Dr. J. F. Yarbrough of Columbia, Alabama, was the first man on his feet. Operator of a pellagra hospital and a strong believer in the use of drugs in treating the disease, Yarbrough called Goldberger's diet treatment "unfortunate," and his abandonment of drugs "nothing short of calamity." Dr. Seale Harris of Atlanta also condemned diet treatment of pellagra. It was too complicated a disease for such simple measures. What about patients who come for treatment in a greatly debilitated state? he asked. Would Goldberger advise only peas and pot liquor? "The results of such prescribing has filled our asylums to overflowing. . . . our cemeteries are blooming as do fields of grain after beneficient summer showers."

Hayne was still angry. He could not again complain about sensational news coverage, but he could and did complain about "diet" treatment. Were diet alone enough, he said, there would be no deaths in pellagra hospitals. A Dallas physician argued that Goldberger's experiments with filth proved nothing, except that pellagra was not directly transmissible from one person to another. What about intermediate carriers? He thought pellagra could originate in the same way as hookworm disease, through larva in the soil. Even James Woods Babcock, whom Goldberger had numbered among his adherents, blamed pellagra on alcohol and talked of finding "hereditary pellagrins at least to the second generation."

Goldberger had his defenders at the Atlanta meeting, and he had an additional advantage he had not had at Dallas the year before: he was there and could defend himself. One physician from Florida termed it unfortunate that one should read "a paper as able as Goldberger's and have it received in such a manner." Another from New Orleans thought all volunteers in the experiment should be awarded gold medals. Goldberger spoke only briefly in his own behalf, but his words were rapier-edged. The mere statement of one's belief in this, that or the other thing about pellagra is a sort of confession of faith, he said: "In my judgment a confession of faith is not debatable."[43] Armed with facts, he made his final thrust at the "impressionistic school" of pellagra research.

Goldberger had hoped to silence the infectionists, but he did not. After the Atlanta meeting, the opposition quieted down a bit but it did not go away. Some months later, MacNeal of the Thompson–McFadden Commission objected in print to Goldberger's transmissibility study, charging that the study proved nothing. If Goldberger really wanted to prove that pellagra was not transmissible, he would have used women aged twenty to forty-five or children aged two to ten, groups much more susceptible to the disease than healthy vigorous men. Goldberger had proved only that men in the more active period of life were quite refractory to the disease.[44]

There were others who also continued to talk about the possibility of pellagra's being contagious. William Petersen, writing in *JAMA* more than a year after the filth experiment, suggested that with increasing migration of Negroes from the South to the North pellagra would increase there. The possibility was not excluded in pellagra that some toxic product was involved or that it was caused by some specific organism not yet isolated.[45] The Pellagra Commission of the National Medical Association stated flatly in 1918 "that pellagra is a communicable and therefore, preventable disease, is abundantly evident to any one open to conviction." It suggested that poor sanitation was directly responsible and that prevention of pellagra, like yellow fever, depended on an inoculating agent.[46]

Goldberger's work was not attacked in a large comprehensive work on pellagra by the Atlanta physician Henry F. Harris published in 1919. Instead, his work was ignored. Harris, credited with spotting the first case of pellagra in the South in 1902, dedicated his book to "master pellagralogists," the Italians Gaetano Strambio and Michael Gherandini, "whose unsurpassed genius excite equally our wonder and admiration." Harris was a convert to the old Italian idea that pellagra was associated with eating maize. The first generation of maize eaters are not affected by pellagra, he suggested, but the poison in them was transmitted to their descendants, becoming more pronounced with each generation.[47]

Harris's book did not deal at all with work done by Americans in the previous decade because, he explained, the great bulk of American literature dealt with subjects and presented views long ago suggested by foreign writers. Harris did praise Babcock for his work and cited as important articles and brochures by twenty-seven other Americans, but Goldberger was not included.[48] The only reference to his work was the inclusion of two of his articles in the bibliography.

If Goldberger was often criticized and occasionally ignored by doctors of the South, and if his educational campaign to change the three-M diet of the region only inched along, he could comfort himself with the knowledge that others working in the new field of nutrition appreciated his work. Success of the prison experiment in 1915 brought praise from Reid Hunt of Harvard Medical School who nominated Goldberger for the Nobel Prize on the basis of his work in typhus, measles, and pellagra. Allan J. McLaughlin, commissioner of health for Massachusetts, wrote his congratulations and called Goldberger America's "foremost figure" in preventive medicine. Elmer V. McCollum wrote that he was "fully convinced" Goldberger was right in interpreting the etiology of pellagra and congratulated him on the thoroughness of his investigations.

In a brief pre-Christmas trip to New York in 1916, Goldberger called on Professor Graham Lusk of Cornell University, an authority on nutrition. They had a long talk and when Goldberger rose to leave, the professor said "I want to say that I have the highest regard for the work you have been doing." Lusk thought it so convincing and conclusive that he used it in the new edition of his work on nutrition, barely giving the infectious idea any notice at all. If a man like Lusk was convinced, thought Goldberger, why worry about such men as Hayne and MacNeal?

In a broad expansive mood he sent Christmas cards to all his friends, including the children at the three orphanages where he had worked, those young friends who so early had boosted his spirits by promptly getting well under his care.[49]

5

A Tale of
Seven Villages

IN THE MONTHS THAT FOLLOWED, Goldberger warded off his critics with one hand and pursued a positive program of research with the other. He suspected that the pellagra-producing three-M diet was not so much a matter of preference as one of economic necessity, but he needed statistical proof. In 1916 he launched an important community study, which was to prove that pellagra was dependent on diet, that diet was determined by economics, and that the economics of the South was determined by its one-crop system. In the next five years, Goldberger was physician, civil engineer, and detective rolled into one.

The most important question to be settled was the relationship of diet to disease. With his associates, Goldberger designed a survey of seven mill villages in South Carolina to find out exactly what the people in these communities ate and how many of them had pellagra. He believed that those marked by the red butterfly would be the same ones who lived on the three-M diet.

Surveys by the Thompson–McFadden Commission in these villages had not measured up to Goldberger's own rigid standards. He found flaws in them, and said so. The commission assumed too much. It was not enough merely to determine roughly how often a particular food was served and then check this against the incidence of pellagra. Thompson–McFadden found that fresh meat had no preventive value because the fewest pellagrins were found among those who never ate fresh meat at all. But the commission made no effort to determine if these pellagra-free, nonmeat eaters had been drinking milk or eating beans and peas.[1] Goldberger thought this was the commission's first mistake. It erred again when it failed to take into account the seasonal nature of the disease, and it erred once more when it took information from households and applied it to individuals. This could not be done; it involved "a confusion of ideas."[2]

His own study was carefully planned to make accurate observations on the diet, economic conditions, and sanitary environment of the area. Associated with him in the work were George A. Wheeler, who had worked with him in the prison experiment, and Edgar Sydenstricker, a PHS economist who was later to become a leading figure in public health. Collection of data began in the spring of 1916 in seven cotton-mill villages in northwestern South Carolina, the same area where local initiative had secured the government Pellagra Hospital when private funds for the study of the disease were exhausted. All were distinct isolated communities made up almost exclusively of cotton-mill employees. Each had 500 to 800 inhabitants, mostly of Anglo-Saxon stock. Only families in roughly the same economic bracket were studied. Mill officials, store managers, and the few Negroes who lived there were not included.[3] Although PHS canvasses, like those of the Thompson–McFadden Commission, collected information on much more than diet, the information they gathered on food bought and consumed was tabulated and published first. The results were all that Goldberger could have wished.

Basic to the study was accurate information on how many

cases of pellagra existed in these seven communities. Working with the permission of mill owners and operatives, Wheeler began a house-to-house canvass in April 1916. On his rounds, he went into every home in every community every two weeks from mid-April through the end of the year. At first people were reluctant to speak of any suspected pellagra, but gradually their reserve disappeared. Wheeler went at different times of the day in order to see personally as many people in each family as possible. He called at noon, on Saturdays, on half-holidays. He checked children coming and going from school or at recess. He went to the mill during working hours to check on suspected cases, and he sought the aid of local physicians in seeking out pellagrins. More than fifty doctors cooperated with him, but they found many fewer cases than Wheeler did. To avoid error, pellagra was carefully defined. Only those patients with a symmetrical dermatitis were counted.[4]

Surveyors working with Wheeler were not content merely to take a person's word for what he had eaten. Instead, they kept a record of the diet of every household for a fifteen-day period during the weeks just before the pellagra season was expected to be at its height. The village stores supplied a record of all food purchased by mill workers or by their families. Enumerators went to every house to find out how many members were in each family, their age and sex, and to determine how much food they purchased from other sources and how much they raised at home. Except for fresh milk, butter, eggs, and meat, little came from any place other than the company stores.[5] Like the coal miners of Kentucky, who had been quizzed several years earlier about their eating habits, these mill workers lived out of paper sacks.

The results were revealing. In households where there was pellagra, the diet included twice as much grits, a fourth more salt pork, and more jelly, jam, and sweet potatoes than did the diet in households where there was none. More important, these same families consumed only four-tenths as much fresh milk, half as much canned milk and fresh meat, and a fifth as much cheese as their healthier neighbors.[6] The relationship of milk to pellagra was most striking. In households where there was less than one quart of milk per person for the fifteen-day period, the incidence of the disease was more than three times larger than in those where there was more milk. Only 3 percent of the families that owned cows had pellagra; 10 percent of the other families were affected. In two-thirds of the households surveyed, there was less than a pound of meat for each person for the two-week period. Nearly all the households with one or more cases of pellagra came from this group. On the other hand, corn seemed to have nothing to do with the disease. Corn-meal was used as freely by one group as another. Neither did the use of dried beans and peas seem to have any effect. Gold-berger had to admit that his earlier observation on the importance of beans was not confirmed.[7]

The dietary survey tied pellagra to food lacking in nutritive value, but it also pointed the way toward a new search which would eventually pinpoint the exact dietary fault. Nutrition research was sufficiently advanced so that Goldberger could narrow the possibilities down to four. There could be something wrong with the protein supply; not all protein was the same, and that from cereals might not be as effective in preventing disease as that from an animal source. There might be an inadequate supply of some vitamin. Fat-soluble A was essential to growth and good vision; water-soluble B could prevent beriberi. Pellagra might be caused by the absence of either a fat- or a water-soluble vitamin. Or there might be a defective mineral supply in the diet. Workers in nutrition had known since the late nineteenth century that certain minerals were essential for life. It could be one of these.[8]

Meanwhile, confirmation of the accuracy of the dietary theory came from two other sources. Wheeler located pellagra cases high in the mountains of Yancey County, North Carolina, at an altitude once thought to be pellagra-proof. The victims there had seldom been more than a few miles from home and had never had contact with pellagrins, but they had been living without meat and milk. From a PHS laboratory came further proof. Monkeys and rats fed an all-vegetable diet showed the extensive degeneration of nerve tissues common to that of pellagrins.[9]

With mounting evidence that pellagra was dependent on diet, it became obvious that there must be something vastly different in the diets of the North and the South. Early in the century, a Yankee gentlewoman who sought various factory jobs in order to see what the life of the working-class woman was really like, described the meals that were set before her in a boarding house in a Southern cotton-mill town. At noon there was a pan of salt pork and another of grease-swimming spinach. For supper there was a platter of fish, another of salt pork, and a dish of hominy. The people she met in the village commented that she must have been used to having good food. Unlike the mill hands, her skin was not sallow, pale, and sickly.[10] A few years later, the British Board of Trade looked into the cost of living in American towns and discovered a striking difference in the diet of the North and the South. Southern families ate much more wheat bread and flour, more molasses and syrup, twice as much bacon and ham, and twice as much lard. On the other hand, they had a low consumption of proteins. Whereas beef and milk were important in the North, salt-hog products and lard were the mainstay of the South.[11]

If Southerners were eating the same foods they had always eaten but had become ill in the twentieth century, there was speculation that some change had happened in one of the basic items of food. Carl Voegtlin, the PHS's vitamin enthusiast, investigated bread and found it wanting. It was not as nourishing as it had been forty years before.

Voegtlin and two associates presented their case against modern-day bread in a sensational article, "Bread as Food," published in *Public Health Reports.*[12] Bread, they said, was a casualty of modern milling. White flour, so much prized by housewives as superior, was instead a distinctly inferior product. Made entirely of but one part of the grain—the starchy endo-sperm—it did not contain the same nutritive value it had when it included the germ and bran as well. The modern roller-mill, introduced in the United States in 1878, had definitely changed the food value of this staple article of the diet. Highly milled flour and cornmeal kept better than whole-grain type but con-tained less protein, ash, and fat than old-fashioned products. More important, highly milled products contained fewer vita-mins, or "certain essential accessory food substances," which were located in the outer layers of the grain and perhaps in the germ.[13]

Changing of the milling process also changed the methods of cooking bread, and Voegtlin and his associates found this new method detrimental. Good cooks soon learned that the new meal, mixed only with salt and water, did not yield a bread of the same lightness as old-fashioned waterground meal, so artificial leavening was added. Baking soda became very popular. It made the bread rise nicely, but it left a strong alkali destruc-tive to vitamins. If buttermilk were used in the bread instead of water, this alkalinity was counteracted, but, as the authors observed in the Spartanburg area, ignorance and inability to get buttermilk often kept this from being done.

Baking soda had still another use in Southern cooking, which showed slight regard for vitamins. Added to beans and other vegetables, it softened them so that they cooked more rapidly, but at the same time, soda had a "greater or less destructive action . . . on vitamines of the beans." It was an expensive time-saver for the person who doubled as family cook and mill worker. Dinner hours at the mills invariably were short, seldom more than thirty minutes. People bolted their food. Theirs was an easy diet to eat on the run. As much as three-fourths of it consisted of biscuits and corn bread.[14]

Reaction to the "Bread As Food" article was swift. The day after it was published, the editor of *Northwestern Miller* tele-graphed the Surgeon General to protest against a "vicious, untrue and wholly unjust attack upon the milling industry." Millers were particularly angry over the yellow journalism twist newspapers gave the article. *The New York Globe* used it as the basis of an attack on all patent flour. The newspaper called it a "debranned, degerminated, demineralized, and debased product which is converted into the broken staff of life, against which the government at last issues warning." Another miller, irate over what he called a "sensational, half-baked article" attributing pellagra to the milling industry, said that even "Dr. [Harvey] Wiley in his palmiest days never hurled this javelin."[15]

Millers had a chance to defend their rights in a hearing before the Secretary of the Treasury in mid-July 1916, and the PHS agreed that, in future publications, it would consult millers before it presented its views on technical features of milling. But attacks on modern milling continued. *The Daily News* of Chicago criticized the quality of bread furnished American armies as inadequate and unfit. Production of highly milled flour dropped nearly 25 percent within a few months, and millers claimed they were hard hit financially. The PHS protested that millers had misinterpreted "Bread As Food," that the paper was not designed as an attack on white bread. It was instead a warning for those people who lived on a largely carbohydrate diet that the probability of pellagra was greater if their bread was made from highly milled flour than it was when made from whole grain.[16]

It was the actual shortage of a good variety of food in the South that was the basic problem. Food people needed simply was not available to those with low incomes. Food production in the South, especially of beef and other animal protein food, lagged behind the rest of the country. Distribution was also poor. As a rule, lean meat was not sold in Southern industrial towns, and, when it was, prices were higher than in the North and Midwest. In some rural districts of Alabama, doctors testified that people not only had pellagra but actually went hungry. Even in cities the size of Spartanburg, there was a shortage of meat. In 1914 practically no meat was shipped into Spartan-burg County by Western packers, and there were no cold-storage facilities there. All meat came from a single slaughterhouse, which sold no more meat in 1914 than it had when there were 20,000 fewer people in the county. A Georgia survey showed the average farm home produced for each member less than two ounces of butter and three eggs a week, only a gill of milk a day, and one-third of a hog, one-tenth of a beef and one-hundredth of a sheep a year.[17]

In mill districts, workers supplemented their food supplies with produce from gardens, which more than a third of the families cultivated. About half as many kept a few chickens, and a few families kept pigs, which were permitted to roam at large through the streets. Earlier in the century, it had been quite common for mill workers to own a cow, but this was increasingly prohibited for sanitary reasons. But all of these makeshift methods of supply were inadequate to cope with the problem of a basic shortage. By 1915 a trend toward crop diversi-fication and toward more beef and milk production had begun, but the shift was not fast enough. As an emergency solution to the South's basic food problem, the Public Health Service suggested raising rabbits. They required no expensive breeding stock, were easily fed, and grew rapidly; they could be killed and dressed at home and eaten the same day so that they re-quired no ice.[18]

The year 1917 was one of the busiest of Goldberger's life. Backed by a $25,000 appropriation from the Public Health Service, he expanded his community study that year from seven villages to twenty-four. One-sixth of the total mill population of South Carolina was under constant scrutiny. Goldberger wanted to establish the significance of age, sex, and race to pellagra and the disease's relationship to geographic, sanitary, and economic conditions. Goldberger and Wheeler were in charge of the study, which again was carried out with the cooperation of state and local health officials, mill owners, store managers, and mill workers. Their staff included two statisticians—Sydenstricker and Wilford I. King—and a field corps of six physicians and a sanitary engineer. Every house in all twenty-four villages was visited every two weeks. The staff asked many personal questions ranging from age and income to what people had in the pantry. It was not an easy job.[19]

Investigators had a hard time getting in the door, and, once inside, their job was a ticklish one. Sometimes they used candy bars and chewing gum to make allies of the children and thus gain an entrance into the house. It took real skill, however, to get answers to their questions. Many people did not want to answer such personal inquiries. Their reticence was natural, and the situation was complicated by the scare of World War I. There was so much talk of German spies that every stranger in the mill villages was immediately under suspicion.[20]

Goldberger was almost constantly on the scene keeping a close check on the work. He described junior officers working under him as "young and more or less frivolous fellows" whom he had to look after and keep up to the mark. Successful outcome of the whole investigation depended on their efficiency. He and Wheeler were out with them every minute they could spare. Always on the move, Goldberger saw plenty of pellagra. By late March he predicted there would be a great deal of it that year. By April there were a "fair number of cases," and in May he could report pellagra was "coming very definitely." Prospects were for "a heavy crop of this reaction to want."[21]

Goldberger was amazed and appalled at the life he saw in these twenty-four villages. He found the pitiful poverty of many people too hard to describe: "I doubt if they are any worse off in Belgium. Some day this will be realized and something done to correct it." He estimated 10 percent or more of the families had at least one case of pellagra, and the horror of it oppressed him. "If we had that much typhoid the militia would probably be called out."[22]

Nothing of what Goldberger and coworkers saw appeared

in the local press, and probably few people outside the villages knew what he was doing. He wanted it that way. A brief story announcing that field investigations. of pellagra were being expanded appeared in the *Spartanburg Journal* on New Year's Day, 1917, and then nothing more. Field workers were instructed not to talk to anybody in town about what they were doing. Publicity would likely break up the work, Goldberger thought. " 'Mum' is the word," he wrote home.[23]

The highlight of Goldberger's summer was the visit of Dr. David Edsall of Harvard University, an authority on occupational diseases. He came South as an admitted skeptic, but he left a believer. As Goldberger put it, he "came to scoff and remained to pray." Before his visit to ten cotton-mill villages, the Pellagra Hospital, and the Georgia Sanitarium, Edsall thought that pellagra, like typhoid, could be attributed to poor sanitation. When he left the South four or five days later, he had changed his mind. Winning so important a convert boosted Goldberger's spirits and encouraged all those engaged in the tedious rounds of house-to-house checks.[24]

Professor Edsall, more impressed than even Goldberger realized, sent a glowing report to the Surgeon General about his visit. Goldberger's three years of experiments and institutional studies, he said, made "unconvincing and well-nigh untenable" any arguments that pellagra was infectious and furnished the "most impressive evidence" that the disease was probably of dietetic origin. All he needed to be wholly convinced was for a few remaining points to be cleared up. What was responsible for the striking incidence of the disease? Why did some villages show a curious freedom from it some years? Why were there occasional cases among people with a generous and varied diet available?[25]

Edsall would not have to wait long for his answers. Meanwhile, he called Goldberger's investigation the most important work he had seen in years. Information it yielded about pellagra would be but a fraction of its true worth for it was a pioneer in the new field of social medicine: "As an example of the study coincidentally of the sanitary, the sociologic, the economic and other important factors influencing disease . . . this is so far as I know, a unique study." He complimented Goldberger and his workers for the care and patience they used in gathering information, which would be quite as valuable in a social and economic way as in a medical way: "This study sets standards that will be very welcome and helpful at this time when the social and economic relations of medicine are becoming clearly recognized."[26]

Goldberger was not the first to recognize the social and economic implications of pellagra, but he was the first to gather enough facts so that the ancient connection of the disease with poverty would be more than a surmise. Rudolph Virchow, a German liberal "Forty-eighter" and long-time champion of social medicine, had observed in the mid-nineteenth century that pellagra resulted from the miserable condition of the people. In the United States, from the time the first case was spotted in 1902, "poverty and pellagra" were linked. By the spring of 1916, when the results of Goldberger's work at the orphanages and the prison experiment were well known, writers in popular magazines pointed out that for all practical purposes the Southern states had control of the disease in their own hands. Pellagra was not the only disease, of course, linked to the economy of a section. Before Goldberger made his survey in the South, the Public Health Service had conducted an industrial study of garment workers in the Pittsburgh area and found that tuberculosis occurred most often among the lowest paid and the least regularly employed people. So much interest was created in this study that in 1916 state health officers endorsed principles of a government health insurance program.[27] But Goldberger's study was unique. Edsall was right about that.[28]

At the end of 1917, field investigations were reduced to a more manageable six villages, and the long process of analyzing the data began. From stacks of cards, a community picture of disease began to emerge, which was at once both better and worse than had been supposed. Pellagra was less severe but far more prevalent than doctors had thought. In the twenty-four villages surveyed in 1917, there were just under fifty-one cases for every thousand people. Only one pellagrin in six ever consulted a doctor, so if physicians sometimes insisted that pellagra was not very widespread, or indeed, occasionally boasted they had never seen a case, they had good reason. Pellagrins did not often call a doctor, because most of them were not very sick, and besides, they did not have the money. A telltale eruption on a child's hand to an ignorant, poverty-stricken parent was not of enough consequence to seek professional help.[29]

One of the most striking facts to emerge from the data was that pellagra was primarily a disease of children. Two-thirds of all cases occurred among children aged two to fifteen. This had not been recognized before because no one had so consciously sought out all these young, but not very sick, victims. Their cases were too mild to excite much attention. The next hardest hit group was comprised of women aged twenty to fifty. There were twenty times as many women affected as there were men in roughly this same age group. Curiously, after the age of fifty, the incidence of pellagra in women dropped progressively with age, while, in men, it rose sharply after forty. There were as many as two to six times more cases than doctors had estimated, but there were not nearly so many fatalities as had once been believed. Allowing for a margin of error, the fatality rate was not more than 3 percent.[30]

Goldberger had an explanation both for the age and sex distribution and for the low fatality rate. He suggested that adolescents (those over fifteen) and men under forty were relatively immune because, as wage earners, they were not only given favorable consideration at the dinner table but they had pocket money and could buy food outside the home. Another possibility was that women had different physiological requirements, that they needed more of some nutritive substance. He attributed the low fatality figures to the completeness of his data (his investigators had overlooked fewer cases) and to the more effective treatment that was available to pellagrins by 1917.[31]

Goldberger was fascinated by the striking seasonal incidence of pellagra. It flared up so suddenly in the spring and subsided so abruptly in the summer he thought it a "remarkable phenomenon." To him, it suggested an annually recurring factor operating within wide geographical limits. Just such a factor he found in the seasonal variation in diet. Pellagra appeared in the spring after a prolonged period of poor diet; it disappeared after the summer months when much better food, such as vegetables and milk, was available even to the poor. In those households where the diet was never very good, even in summer, pellagrins did not have time to recover fully from an attack before the long hard winter of even leaner fare began. In these cases, a recurrence was likely very early the following spring.[32]

The South Carolina survey not only supported Goldberger's dietary theory, but showed forcefully that the infectious theory was wrong in spite of all the Thompson–McFadden Commission said to the contrary. The commission issued its final report in the fall of 1916, stating emphatically that the disease was infectious and the only way to combat it was with efficient sewage disposal systems. It based its case on an intensive three-year study of Spartan Mills, South Carolina, which it called one of the "worst pellagra districts in the South." Scores of people suffered attacks of pellagra each year so long as there was no sewer system, but as soon as this defect was remedied, pellagra virtually disappeared. There were still recurrences, but only one new case. The commission thought the evidence conclusive.[33]

Goldberger quickly demolished the commission's findings. There was no reduction of pellagra in Spartan Mills, his studies showed. The disease was at least as prevalent there as in a nearby village with the crudest, most insanitary methods. It was the difference in income that mattered. When this was recorded on maps of villages, it was obvious why the Thompson–McFadden Commission had gone astray. Higher-income families were grouped in that part of the village closest to the residence of foremen and other officials. Transients or "rolling stones" who made much less money were grouped in another part of town. It was in these sections that most cases of pellagra were found. It was only accidental if this disease and insanitary conditions occurred at the same place. Both were the offspring of poverty.[34]

The case for the dietary theory was so convincing that even the *Southern Medical Journal* published an editorial accepting it as a matter of course and admonishing doctors to take notice. It had been but three years since that same journal had laughed at the idea. With important men like Edsall convinced, Goldberger thought the matter settled. "All the pop-guns are at once silenced!"[35]

What silenced them was the thorough way in which Goldberger and his associates tied pellagra to poverty. The connection could not be denied. For statistician Edgar Sydenstricker, this was the second time around. He had done the first important economic study on pellagra in 1915 and presented his findings at the National Association for the Study of Pellagra in Columbia, South Carolina, the same meeting at which Goldberger had described the success of dietary treatment in Georgia and Mississippi. Sydenstricker suggested the alarming increase in pellagra that year might be due to the rising cost of food in wartime. With nine-tenths of Southern mill workers earning less than $7 a week, any increase in the cost of food could be disastrous. Since 1904, while wages advanced only 25 percent, retail food prices went up 60 percent. To maintain the same diet in 1913 as in 1900, the average workingman's family in the South Atlantic states needed $155 more a year, and, in the South Central states, it needed an additional $192 a year. Since wages had not gone up that much, it was "impossible to assume that this diet has been maintained."[36]

Sydenstricker's report on pellagra offered a new insight into life in Southern mill villages, a subject of inquiry since the great influx of people into these villages from the rural areas began about the turn of the century. The most comprehensive study was included in the government's investigation on the condition of women and child wage earners.[37] Shorter, less systematic investigations, many in the form of exposés, appeared regularly in national magazines. The "people of the cotton mill" became a favorite topic during these years. Muckrakers did not have to look hard to find something wrong with life in the mill villages. Long hours, low pay, filth, and the sheer monotony of life lent themselves well to the muckrakers' cause. Yet, occasionally, there was a writer who pointed out the somber truth that life in the mill villages, bad as it was, was actually better than many workers had known on the farm. Even on low mill wages, some of them had more real money than they had ever seen in their lives. If they encountered pellagra in the villages, it was no stranger to them. It was a spectre many had already met on the farms from which they fled.[38]

If muckrackers were fascinated by conditions in the mills, most South Carolinians were not. By 1916 it was obvious that the textile industry of the state was coming into the hands of outsiders. What happened in the mill villages then, including a high increase in disease, was of little concern to nonmill workers. Any problem in the mills was of interest only to two parties—the laborers and the owners—and South Carolinians in other callings had only an indefinite and vague interest in it. Only occasionally was the plight of the workers recognized by South Carolinians. *The State* in Columbia urged mill workers to unionize in 1915 so that they might be freed from the helplessness and hopelessness that depressed them.[39]

In the summer of 1917 Goldberger, an outsider, was worried about the mill workers. He was afraid the crowding of soldiers into Spartanburg and the consequent soaring of prices would make the mill hand's lot even more difficult than it already was. With fresh vegetables, milk, and eggs very hard to get

and everybody living out of tin cans, he thought life in Spartanburg must have been a little like that of Western gold mining
camps. He wondered how the poor people were going to survive.[40] This time he was worried unnecessarily. War prosperity
made prices rise, but so did wages, and mill workers were better
off than they had ever been in their lives. Pellagra began to
disappear.

The war did Goldberger a favor. For a while, it not only
cut down the number of pellagrins, but spurred on active interest
in nutrition. Southerners chanted Herbert Hoover's slogan "Food
Will Win The War" along with the rest of the nation, and
a good many took it to heart. Some Southern farmers plowed
land already planted with cotton and put in foodstuffs, and
there was much more interest in protective foods. Good nutrition, about which much of the public had been only vaguely
aware, was pushed in the name of patriotism.[41]

Emphasis on a better diet was especially marked among
Negroes. The Messengers, a national organization of black men
and women, carried the message of the Food Administration
to their race. "Hoe the world to victory," they said, and their
message fell on receptive ears. Negro women in South Carolina
canned nearly 21,000 quarts of fruits and vegetables in 1917
in spite of wild rumors that the government planned to confiscate
all canned fruit. A professor at Tuskegee Institute in Alabama
credited the Food Administration propaganda with awakening
in a few months more interest among Negroes in home economics
than formal educational facilities had been able to do in years.
For the first time, blacks became interested in diet, economy,
saving, and food production. W. E. B. Du Bois said the food
conservation program of World War I was a blessing: "There
is no doubt but what Americans and colored Americans in particular eat too much. They do not choose the most nourishing
foods and often they choose food which is wasteful and harmful.
Here now in the stress of war comes a chance to correct bad
habits."[42]

In Spartan Mills village, one of those included in Goldberger's survey, mill officials offered to plow all garden spots and furnish seed free to mill workers in the spring of 1917. The offer was made in view of the high cost of living that year and in response to appeals from the government and the chamber of commerce to plant gardens. As part of the war effort, the Public Health Service launched an extensive publicity campaign on diet and pellagra and distributed thousands of pamphlets. State health departments hired their first nutritionists in 1917. South Carolina's Senator "Cotton Ed" Smith maintained his keen interest in agriculture that first wartime spring, too, but he did not urge his constituents to plant gardens. He was in Washington protesting because there were no government ships available to bring millions of dollars of nitrates from Chile. He thought production of corn and cotton could be doubled if only the Chilean nitrates were available.[43]

In spite of progress made during the war, Southern diets continued to be less nutritious than those of other sections. A World War I survey showed that maize composed 23 percent of the total intake of Tennessee and Georgia mountaineers and more than 32 percent of the diet of Southern Negroes, but less than 2 percent of the diet of Northern families in comfortable circumstances. Corn, pork, and syrup, all remnants of a frontier heritage, remained the basic diet of the South.[44]

To the Public Health Service team working in South Carolina, pellagra came to be a symbol of a community's economic well-being, as well as a mark of individual poverty. When times were good, pellagra vanished from a village; when they were bad, it reappeared. Goldberger's study was not a comparison of the rich and the poor. Rather, it was a comparison of the poor with the very poor. The range of income in the families investigated was small. Most had an income of about $700 a year; few had incomes of more than $1,000. The difference was in the number of people, their age, and their sex for which this small amount had to provide.[45]

In the families studied in 1916, PHS workers found a perfect inverse correlation of income and pellagra. For those who had an income of less than $6 per adult male unit for a fifteen-day period, incidence of the disease was just under forty-three cases per thousand population. It dropped steadily with each increase in income until it stood at less than three-and-a-half cases per thousand for those who had $14 or more. Two or more cases per family occurred only in the lower income classes. A check of the pantries showed that the smaller the income, the smaller the supplies of all meat (except salt pork), green vegetables, fresh fruits, eggs, butter, cheese, preserved milk, lard, sugar (including syrup), and canned foods. The smaller the income, the larger the supplies of salt pork and cornmeal.[46]

Incidence of pellagra varied from village to village, being rampant in some and totally lacking in others where people were equally poor. In these cases, the decisive factor was availability of food supplies. A case in point was the village of Inman Mills in Spartanburg County, where more than sixty-four people out of every thousand had pellagra, and the village of Newry in Oconee County where there was not a single case. Both villages had company stores, and, in both, residents also shopped for groceries in adjacent communities. But there was more food available in Newry than in Inman Mills. In Newry a fresh-meat market was open seven days a week all year. Fresh fruits and vegetables were also sold, and the village was a center for marketing produce from nearby farms. Newry was located in an area where raising cotton was less profitable, so farmers put more emphasis on vegetable gardens and on raising cattle, poultry, and milk cows.

The country around Inman Mills, on the other hand, was planted mostly in cotton. There was little truck farming done, few beef cattle were raised, and only enough milk was produced to supply the needs of the farmers. There were no regular peddlers of produce in Inman Mills in 1916, and fresh fruits and vegetables were not often available in the company store.

In Inman Mills, 91 percent of the low income families purchased no milk, butter, eggs, fresh vegetables, fruit, or poultry. In Newry, more than 83 percent of the families purchased at least some of these items, and more than half the families bought milk.[47]

Availability of good food and money enough to buy it were in themselves incapable of preventing pellagra in all cases. The food had to be eaten. Here Goldberger found an explanation for the occasional case of pellagra that appeared among well-to-do families. The fact that pellagra virtually disappeared from those families with incomes as small as $1,000 a year indicated that cases in families with larger incomes were truly exceptional. When they occurred, they could be attributed to eccentricity of taste, a prejudice against some foods, or ill-advised dieting.[48]

Primarily, pellagra was a social and economic problem. It was a "hard times" disease, the natural outcome of a crop failure or a financial depression. That explained the tremendous increase in the number of pellagrins in 1915. The depression, which developed just after the outbreak of war in 1914 when cotton could not be sold, made money short that winter, and pellagra followed like a spring crop. So long as the South depended on a single crop, Goldberger believed there would be pellagra. The failure of the cotton crop, or a sudden drop in price when too much was produced or when markets were lost, upset a perilously balanced economy and took an immediate toll in the health of the people. He believed that any adverse turn in the economy could be used to predict an increase in pellagra the following season.[49]

Just as Goldberger kept his survey out of the local press, he maintained a silence on the relation of pellagra to poverty and the one-crop system. A report of the findings of 1916 on the economic factors of pellagra was not published until 1920, and the complete report of work done over the five-year period did not appear until 1929. Perhaps the reason for silence was that the PHS team did not want to lose the support and backing of local physicians and mill officials. The relationship of pellagra to poverty was to be even more disturbing to the sensitive nerves of the South than the relationship of pellagra to diet had been. Had Goldberger released his findings while the study was still underway, the cooperation he and his field workers had received from the mill operatives in answering hundreds of questions probably would have vanished.

For whatever reason, Goldberger remained silent, and the public remained largely unaware of what he was doing. Almost the only public notice given the association of pellagra with low income was Sydenstricker's paper presented at the Columbia pellagra conference late in 1915. *The State* took due notice of this and commented editorially that it would be better not to have cotton mills than to have diseased mill operatives. Probing further into the problem, *The State* observed that the rural poor, as well as the mill workers, were affected.

> At the bottom of the trouble is the Negro. . . . Unfortunately the great proportion of white people care little how the Negro lives, so long as he furnishes the labor. The wage of the Negro, directly or indirectly, affects the wage scale of every other class of labor in the South. Our commercial fabric and our civilization are built on cheap Negro labor and, of course, we do not escape the evils attendant upon it. Save for the fact that the landless white man cannot always successfully compete with the Negro on the farm, there would be no native cotton mill operatives.
>
> Obviously the only way of improving conditions in the South is to begin at the bottom, and that means that we should train and educate all our people, Negroes and whites, so that they would produce more and earn better wages and be better citizens. So long as we cling to the barbarous notion that Negroes shall be held in ignorance and remain cheap laborers, our poor whites will be dragged down to their economic level. Economic laws draw no color line.[50]

There was no easy answer to the problem of poverty and pellagra. Wilford I. King, who was in immediate charge of the statistical phases of the pellagra investigations, asked the questions: do mill owners have to pay a living wage? Is the employer responsible for employees who are drifters, here today and gone tomorrow? The South had such an oversupply of igno-

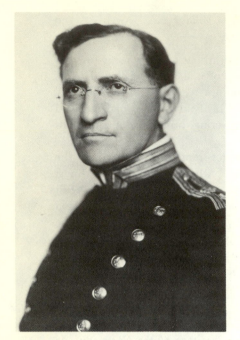

Dr. Joseph Goldberger in his
Public Health Service uniform.

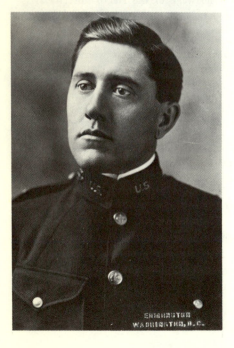

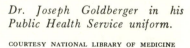

Dr. George A. Wheeler, Goldberger's closest associate, who
worked with him in the prison
experiment and in the South Carolina mill villages.

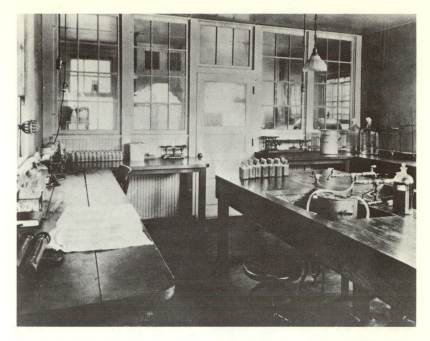

An interior view of the Hygienic Laboratory, research arm of the Public Health Service, around 1902.

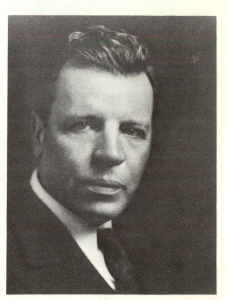

Edgar Sydenstricker, statistician for the pellagra studies in the South Carolina mill villages from 1917 through 1921.

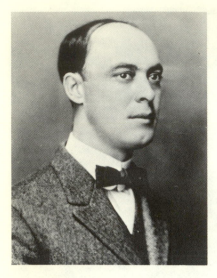

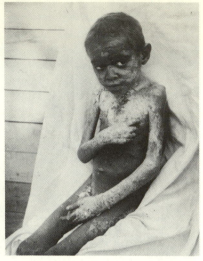

Dr. C. H. Waring, who worked
with Goldberger at the Jackson,
Mississippi, orphanages.

A severe case of pellagra in a
child of about six.

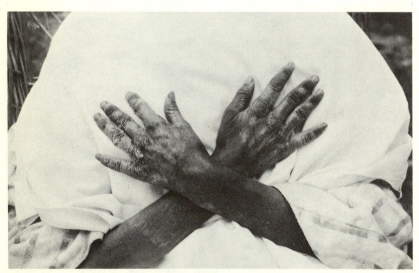

A woman's hands showing the skin lesions of pellagra.

rant and inefficient labor. The problem was bigger than just educating the people in the three R's and on the basic fundamentals of diet. What was needed was the kind of education which would give inspiration and stimulate ambition among the South's poor. This would raise the standard of living, lower the birth rate, decrease the supply of unskilled labor, raise wages, diminish poverty, and, coincidentally, cause the practical disappearance of pellagra.[51]

During the war years and after as Goldberger tramped around the dingy streets of the little cotton-mill villages, checking the people's hands and faces for the ugly red marks of pellagra, and checking endlessly on how much money they made and how they spent it, he pieced together in his mind a picture of how pellagra was an index to the economic well-being of a community, but he told nobody else. The war years were good ones for the people of the mill villages. In April 1920 wages were three-and-a-quarter times as much as they had been in 1916. Food costs had risen, too, but not that much. These were but little more than double the 1916 level. There was still pellagra in the villages, but it was not the ever-present horror it had been. Goldberger made plans to close both the Pellagra Hospital in Spartanburg and the field office there. The PHS team had gathered all the data it needed, and the hospital, set up to make metabolism studies on pellagra, had completed its work. No more patients were admitted to the hospital after July 1, 1920, and the entire operation was closed by the first of the following year.[52]

On closing the hospital, the Spartanburg County Medical Society honored Goldberger and Wheeler at a banquet. "We have met for a funeral and an interment. We are here to bury pellagra," a local physician told the group. Another assured Goldberger and Wheeler that Spartanburg physicians "haven't a thing against you. . . . To come to a town such as ours, to rub up against half a hundred physicians, notoriously cranky and jealous and conceited and opinioned, and yet gain the ill will of none, speaks well indeed for your courtesy and your tact and your diplomacy." Goldberger wished for a dissenter in the group. They could not all be 100 percent believers. He warned that while pellagra had been relieved by prosperity, there was a possibility hard times would make it return. In that event, people would know how to treat the disease. But his warning was swallowed up in the festiveness of the occasion, and, in the press account of the event, it was buried toward the end of a very long story.[53]

Goldberger knew then that trouble was on the way. The price of cotton dropped so quickly in the fall of 1920 that it caught unaware those who somehow thought the golden days of cotton prosperity would last forever. When the time came for tenant farmers and sharecroppers to settle their accounts that fall, they received less than half as much cash as they had recieved in 1919. The price dipped so low that some plantation owners decided to hold their cotton off the market and hope for a better price. Tobacco brought but little more than a third as much as it had brought the year before. The number of farm owners shrank; there were many more mortgages.[54]

In late summer of 1920 Goldberger had gone to Mississippi at the request of the state board of health to investigate an increase in pellagra there. He visited Isola and Holly Bluff and Bentonia and Belzoni in the rich delta region. An overflow of the Yazoo River had covered much of the farming land from late March to the end of May, ruining crops and grazing lands and blocking rail shipments. It was impossible to plant gardens and to bring in perishable food from other areas. Bad as the situation was in 1920, Goldberger thought it would be worse in 1921. Most of the farming was done by renters who had no capital of their own but were furnished essential supplies by the plantation owner or merchant on the basis of crop prospects. The overflow made these dubious. Credit was certain to be tight in the delta region. To tenant farmers, tight credit was but a prelude to illness the next spring.[55]

In the mill villages where Goldberger had spent so much time, the end of wartime prosperity came swiftly. In November 1920, wages dropped, and they continued to fall until they were cut almost in half. The PHS field office in Spartanburg was closed in October. Less than a week after the banquet at which pellagra had been buried with such ceremony, Goldberger asked the Surgeon General to reopen it. The studies from April 1916 until 1920 covered a period of improved economic conditions. The advent of depression provided an opportunity to study the same area under unfavorable conditions. He proposed to limit the study that year to but a single village—Inman Mills—one of the original seven villages surveyed and one that had been under constant scrutiny for five years. Under Wheeler's direction work began again: the house-to-house checks, the visits to the company store and other shops that sold food, the endless questions about what people ate, how much they paid for it, and how much money they had to meet all their expenses. With the Pellagra Hospital closed, the field office took on some of the aspects of a clinic. Patients and local physicians came by often seeking advice and help.[56]

Certainly pellagra had not been "buried," in spite of the fact that in a half-dozen years Goldberger and his associates in the Public Health Service had provided answers to most of the questions of two centuries about the disease. They had learned exactly how to prevent it and how to cure it, and, at the Georgia State Sanitarium, they had begun a systematic search for the mysterious missing quantity in the Southern diet. Their best efforts, however, brought them squarely against a problem far more difficult of solution than the ones they had unraveled in six years of hard work. Pellagra was the fruit of poverty, and for this problem there was no ready answer. There was only Southern pride and anger that it should be mentioned at all. When Goldberger finally mentioned the unmentionable, Southerners became very angry with him indeed.

6

Famine, Plague,
and Furor

MONTHS AFTER Goldberger became aware that pellagra would greatly increase in 1921 and would surely be worse the following year, he broke his self-imposed silence. From a hotel in Union, South Carolina, he wrote a letter that set ever widening waves in motion and broke the calm of a Southern summer. Before their energy was spent, these waves would reach the halls of Congress and the President of the United States.

The letter, sent to the PHS headquarters in Washington, spoke plainly: "For all practical purposes we have in our own country this summer thousands of people who are starving and dying. . . . We are feeding the Near East and the Far East but we are neglecting our own people here at home." Goldberger told how serious he and Wheeler had found the situation in the South Carolina mill village they were studying, and how Edgar Sydenstricker had reported similar distress in Nashville, Tennessee. There was trouble in Mississippi, too, and Goldberger hoped the health officials there, usually cooperative in pellagra work, would again take the lead in awaking public attention to the problem.[1]

Within a few days, his hopes were fulfilled. Dr. W. S. Leathers, executive officer of the Mississippi State Board of Health, requested Surgeon General Hugh Cumming to call a meeting of state health officers and prominent laymen to emphasize the need for proper educational methods to keep pellagra under control.[2]

It was Goldberger who drew up a plan to handle the emergency. Because it was mid-July and too late to take preventive measures, he concentrated on treating the sick. He wanted food, medical and nursing advice for pellagrins, and hospitalization for the more seriously ill. He thought the Red Cross might help. He hoped plantation owners and mill managers would set up clinics through which aid could be dispersed. There must be publicity; people had to be aroused to the current danger and to the more serious threat posed for 1922.

His fear of the worst was not based on mere speculation. In Inman Mills, South Carolina, his surveyors found 31 cases of pellagra in 1921; there had been only 14 the year before. In Mississippi, there were 1,817 new cases in May, almost triple the figure for May 1920. Doctors in Spartanburg and in Memphis reported seeing more pellagrins. The economic pressure felt throughout the South compelled the "utmost economy in household expenditures," Goldberger noted in a memorandum. Tenant farmers were forced to cut down on their food supplies by the merchants, the planter landlords, or the banks who "furnished" them. Reduced wages forced mill workers to the same economy. He doubted if profits for the cheaply produced cotton crop of 1921 would be enough to liquidate the losses from the still unsold expensively produced crop of 1920. Credit was certain to be tighter in 1922 than it was in 1921, and, if so, more pellagra was sure to follow. Most of all, Goldberger wanted to reach planters and tenants to tell them that they must plant food crops on some of their lands. Then, if cotton should fail, the quality of their diet would not depend completely on whatever credit the bankers or merchants could afford. He wanted also to educate people to the necessity of making more food available in small isolated industrial communities. He still advocated owning a cow.[3]

The program began with publicity. If Goldberger remembered the furor created by newspaper coverage of the prison experiment, he apparently did not care if the same thing happened again. The prison experiment publicity had angered only a portion of the medical profession. His new endeavor, reported in newspapers throughout the United States, linked pellagra to the basic poverty of the South and angered laymen and politicians of the region. They resented having the South's poor financial status paraded before the nation. An increase in pellagra was a disgrace that they hotly and persistently denied.

The original story announcing an increase in pellagra in the South showed little restraint. Goldberger wanted publicity and he got it. The story, though emanating from PHS headquarters in Washington, was based on Goldberger's letter from South Carolina and the memorandum he had sent from Mississippi. In that first story the PHS called pellagra one of the "worst scourges known to man," saying that it was making "alarming" headway in the cotton belt and that it was due to "semi-starvation." The story added that pellagra would claim 100,000 victims in 1921, of whom 10 percent, or 10,000, would die. The PHS predicted worse things to come for the enfeebled population in 1922: "While the American people have been spending money lavishly to save the Chinese and Europeans from starvation a veritable famine has been developing in the rural districts of the South, . . . and particularly in those of the cotton belt which stretches from Eastern Texas to the Carolinas. The tenant farmers . . . have been forced by the failure of the cotton market to adopt a starvation diet that is rapidly decimating them." Goldberger was quoted as saying that the situation was worse in Mississippi, in the Memphis, Tennessee, area, and in parts of eastern Texas and the Carolinas. Only the fruit crop had saved Georgia. The program of aid and education outlined in the newspapers was the one he had recommended to the Surgeon General.[4]

Southern newspapers did not give this story much attention, reporting simply that the disease had been "spotted," but the *New York Times* put it on page one.[5] An interested reader was President Warren G. Harding, who promptly asked Surgeon General Cumming for a complete report on the situation in the South and suggestions for proper action. He also asked the American Red Cross for help. The President promised to request legislative action if it should be necessary. He minced no words. The fact that the condition of semifamine was due to economic dislocation following the war did not lessen the concern of the nation. "Famine and plague are words almost foreign to our American vocabulary, save as we have learned their meaning in connection with the afflictions of lands less favored and toward which our people have so many times displayed large and generous charity," he wrote the Surgeon General. The nation could not wait a single day to take action. It must save its own.[6]

The Surgeon General was delighted with the President's letter. He thought it quickly and effectively focused attention on the many different phases of the problem, and he believed it would facilitate federal–state cooperation in solving it. Goldberger was pleased, too, and granted an interview in which he expanded his views on what ought to be done to save the South. The Public Health Service had only $18,000 with which to fight pellagra; it needed $140,000, and this did not include hospitalization or relief supplies for the victims. He wanted to put one pellagra expert in each state, as well as one dietitian and one clinic in every state, which could treat at least one hundred pellagrins each, instruct them on diet, and send them home to instruct their neighbors. These patients could get by on one good meal a day, costing about twenty-five cents each. The real problem, Goldberger pointed out again, was economic: "If economic conditions do not improve I would be loath to prophesy what the 1922 story will be."[7]

He had other ideas about what could be done to help. In addition to the clinics for ambulatory patients and hospital care for the more seriously ill, he suggested that local relief be so organized that those without money or credit could get a minimum supply of essential foods and that more milk, eggs, cheese, lean meats, and vegetables be made available by stimulating local production. Plantation stores and camp commissaries could help by carrying supplies of cheap canned meats and fish.[8]

Goldberger was something of a modern-day Jeremiah, and he proved to be no more popular. Instead of action, he got reaction. It was President Harding's letter that so upset the people of the South. Many Southerners first learned of the pellagra menace when they read the President's "famine and plague" letter, which was given top billing in many newspapers. The protests were not long in coming. One of the first was from Florida promoters who were afraid the blanket indictment against the cotton states would create an unfavorable psychology toward Florida, which did not consider itself part of the cotton belt. Specifically, Floridians were afraid the report would frighten away tourists. Georgia's Senator William J. Harris at once had a conference with Surgeon General Cumming and Goldberger to ascertain the true situation in the South, but was unconvinced by their statistics. Afterward he reported with satisfaction, it was "nothing like the alarming statement first published."[9]

A few groups actually praised the Public Health Service for its timely action and pledged their support, but these were in the minority. At first, the United Daughters of the Confederacy, 100,000 strong, thanked President Harding for his concern over the suffering in the cotton district, but less than a month later, their gratitude turned to anger. They decided that a grave injustice had been done the cotton states by the false reports. "Famine does *not exist* anywhere in the South," the ladies protested, "and we fail to find evidence of a general increase in pellagra."[10]

The rush to get on the anti-PHS bandwagon was reminiscent

of the protest against John D. Rockefeller's million-dollar fight to eradicate hookworm in 1909. Southerners then had felt insulted at the suggestion that people had worms. They resented the Northern press's attempt at humor in talking about the "germ of laziness" and a Methodist bishop had called the Rockefeller gift a "dumdum donation."[11] But the voice of reason eventually prevailed in the hookworm campaign and so it would in the new fight on pellagra, too, but it would take time.

The editor of *The State* in Columbia had been disgusted in 1909 with Southerners who felt themselves "insulted" by Rockefeller's gift: "The intelligent sober men of the South have long ago become wearied and disgusted with this sectional chip that some of our spokesmen insist upon carrying on their shoulders. . . . They are sick of this exploitation of the 'sensitiveness' of a 'proud' people." In 1921, Southerners were still proud and sensitive. *The Greensboro* (North Carolina) *Daily News* predicted correctly that the South's pained astonishment at the discovery of a new wave of pellagra would be exchanged for one of outraged innocence: "Delusions of persecution will begin to arise and be carefully fostered. Somebody in the administration has it in for the South. It will be recalled that the President comes from Ohio, and is therefore, a damyankee, who has probably spent the major portion of his active life devising ways and means of afflicting the South." The editor thought some "super-hearted ex-Confederate" was pretty sure to break loose with a thundering denunciation of the wicked designs of President Harding.[12]

Southern sensitivity, so much a part of the Southern experience it did not have to be explained to anyone south of the Mason-Dixon line, was an enigma to those north of it. Its roots ran deep, back a hundred years to the time when Southerners would brook no criticism of slavery, the "peculiar insitution" which set the South apart from the rest of the nation. Then their defense had been to praise the South as the most perfect civilization the world had ever known. When this perfect civilization was destroyed in the Civil War, the pain of defeat had been somewhat eased by the sentimental glorification of the "lost cause" and by the widespread belief that, given enough time, the South would rise again. The idea of a New South—strong, vigorous, idealistic—was pervasive. Any revelation which cast doubt that the phoenix had indeed risen from the ashes was to be denied. Both hookworm and pellagra cast doubt. Both were symbols of poverty. Both were found among tenant farmers and croppers, classes which had multiplied as Southerners sought a substitute for slave labor, and among mill workers, the cheap labor force without whom the textile industry, hallmark of the New South, could not exist. The Northern press could not understand the almost hysterical denials which President Harding's letter brought forth. "Almost it would seem that they did not wish a fight to be made upon pellagra," a Michigan paper commented, "that they had adopted that disease as something to be quite expected, something indigenous to the South and not to be interfered with."[13] That was not it at all. It was not that pellagra was sacred, but that its existence said too much about the Southern way of life. If only the disease could have been carried by a mosquito!

Politicians who made the political error of expressing concern over the spread of pellagra in the South quickly ate their words and joined those who flailed the Public Health Service. South Carolina's Senator N. B. Dial was among these. He got an unusual amount of attention because President Harding publicly referred to the Senator's concern over pellagra and sent him copies of the famous "famine and plague" letters he wrote the Surgeon General and Red Cross officials. Senator Dial inadvertently stumbled into the national spotlight because of a request he made to the Public Health Service a week before pellagra became such a national issue. Having seen local reports that the disease was increasing, he asked the PHS to take action to prevent its spread and to reopen the hospital at Spartanburg, should that be necessary.[14] He was soon sorry he had ever mentioned it.

The report circulated that it was he who had called President Harding's attention to the pellagra situation in the South and that it was he who had led the Surgeon General to believe that semifamine existed there. The Senator denied it. There was no danger of famine in the South, he insisted with increasing vehemence. All would be well in Dixie were it not for the unjust cotton-futures contract law and the unjust railroad rates, a kind of "thievery," he said, that had the protection of Congress. Insofar as pellagra was concerned, Senator Dial expressed surprise that the Public Health Service had discontinued studying a disease before they had ascertained the cause of it.[15]

His colleague from South Carolina, Congressman James F. Byrnes, was in a more fortunate position. Having never expressed concern about pellagra, it was enough for him to label as an "utter absurdity" reports of famine and plague in South Carolina and to decline in advance a possible offer of Red Cross aid. "We may be over sensitive," he wrote President Harding, "but the average American dislikes to have placed in front of his door a flag indicating the presence of a plague, when . . . there exists within his home nothing to justify that characterization." And, he added, the South disliked being held up as an object of charity and compared with the "unfortunates of other lands." Very angry, Byrnes asked that appropriate action be taken against those officials who had misrepresented the situation and led the President into making the "famine and plague" statement.[16]

Congress became the national forum for debating the slander of the South, beginning the day the President wrote the offending letters. Southern congressmen and senators leaped to defend the honor of the homeland. There was no "grim and gaunt spectre of famine . . . walking abroad in the Empire State of the South," Georgia's Congressman W. C. Wright protested. True, the boll weevil and the drop in the price of cotton from forty-five to ten cents a pound had made times hard, but Georgians could work out their own salvation. As the citizens of one south Georgia city wired Senator Tom Watson, "when this part of Georgia suffers from a famine the rest of the world will be dead." Tennessee, too, boasted of an abundance of food. The state health officer issued an invitation through Senator Kenneth McKellar to all the fearful to come to Tennessee for old-time square meals so they could see how healthy Tennesseans headed off famine. In fact, Tennessee stood ready to ship beef, pork, poultry, and milk to her poorer neighbors in the North just as soon as Congress stabilized the markets. Congressmen from Florida and Oklahoma insisted that their states, too, would ship food to other states if freight rates were not prohibitory. Oklahoma branded the famine reports as "malicious propaganda."[17]

Thus was the honor of the South upheld in the halls of Congress. Under the guidance of an "All-Wise Being," Georgia's Congressman Wright predicted, the South would be saved: "Cotton will once more be enthroned as King, and the fair Southland will again come into her own, blossom as the rose, and her people will be contented and happy."[18] There were some who thought that if the Congressmen spent more time working for the South and less time defending its sacred honor that all the South would profit. Specifically, cotton growers and manufacturers wanted more liberal credit. They asked that the Federal Reserve Board lower its rediscount rates or that the War Finance Corporation be reinstated. Only this, they said, would secure the needed relief for rehabilitation of life in the cotton belt.[19]

Southern political leaders, almost as one, denied that pellagra was increasing, and from the health departments of Tennessee, Louisiana, Alabama, North Carolina, Virginia, and Georgia came echoes of these denials. A few health officers not only denied that there was any more disease than usual but even said it was decreasing. Actually, most state health officers did not know what the true situation was in their own states. Pellagra was not a reportable disease in many states, including

Georgia, Louisiana, North Carolina, and Texas. Health officers could deny an increase in pellagra, but they could not prove it. The health officer from Arkansas admitted that there seemed to be more cases than usual, but that certainly no state of semi-famine existed. Hayne, South Carolina's peppery health officer, admitted that there had been an increase in the number of pellagra deaths, but he called the Washington report of a sharp increase an attempt to cast reflections on the South. The strangest denial of all came from Leathers, of Mississippi, who had but shortly before urged that a conference on pellagra be called. Leathers, perhaps to save face at home, called the report of more pellagra "absolutely ridiculous. . . . It is preposterous. Of course, there are some isolated cases in which families may be in want, but that is also found in New York City. Evidently the alarm of a menace is a result of making a mountain out of a molehill." The Public Health Service was not really surprised at the denials. Telegraphic inquiries at the departments indicated that they did not know what the conditions were. Federal officials reasoned that state health authorities had to deny the existence of pellagra lest their departments be given a "black eye."[20] They did not want the reports to get out, so they denied them altogether.

The pellagra scare quickly spread from the realm of health to those of business and politics. The Georgia Senate passed a resolution denouncing the report of a pellagra epidemic as "damning." The Atlanta Chamber of Commerce complained that the report was unwarranted by facts and was likely to prove another serious blow to the South. The governor of Alabama suspected that the South was being slurred as part of a propaganda campaign for some other section, and *The Atlanta Constitution* called the report of semifamine conditions "bosh and poppycock." Businessmen of Memphis, Tennessee, feared the President's action would be disastrous to business interests. People in Spartanburg, South Carolina, thought it necessary to explain that just because the government's Pellagra Hospital had been located in their city, Spartanburg was not the seat of an outbreak of the disease. There was no poverty in the cotton-mill villages in the area, they protested. The people were paid good wages. Only ignorance kept them from buying food that would give them a well-balanced diet.[21] Almost half a century later, when reports came out of Beaufort that people were hungry, South Carolinians again denied it. Impossible, they said.

Indignantly, the South spurned charity. The associate publisher of the *Columbia* (S.C.) *Record* wired Congressman Byrnes that South Carolina was able and willing to look after any "derelicts" of its own and would spurn attempts to make the state a charity ward: "The President has been woefully misled and we are now striving to find out why our senators wobbled into the fog." Small wonder that Senator Dial was defending himself in Congress. Times were hard, the *Memphis Commercial Appeal* commented editorially, but the South would bear its burdens in a "manly and courageous way"; it would never be a charity patient on the nation. This newspaper scored the government's "new-fangled experts" who blamed pellagra on a diet of salt pork, corn bread, and molasses. Obviously, it said, these experts did not know that for a half century and more the Southern Negro had lived and grown strong on such a diet. From Alabama, heart of Dixie, came a second to this idea: "Don't the dern fools [government experts] know that for four long years the Confederate soldiers had mighty little else to eat except swine bosom, corn pone and molasses, and there never was a case of pellagra heard of in the army?"[22] Confederate soldiers may or may not have had pellagra. The disease was not recognized then. But certainly, thousands of blacks had it in 1921. In a state like Mississippi where the number of pellagrins was known, blacks outnumbered whites.

To prove that there was no starvation in the South, it became almost standard procedure to recite the bounty of the section. This was especially true in Georgia, which prided itself on increasing diversification of agriculture, despite what Congressman Wright said in Washington about cotton always being king. "We are quite cured of all cotton," the editor of *The Augusta Chronicle* commented. The South had been foolish enough to plant cotton to its financial hurt, but it was learning its lesson. "Rations Plentiful," *The Savannah Morning News* proclaimed in headlines stretching across the page. Money might be scarce, but there were full plates in south Georgia. Indeed, the low price of cotton seemed to have helped the food situation, *The Morning News* continued. More food crops were being grown than ever before. The situation seemed so good in Burke County that the editor of the local paper wrote with tongue-in-cheek that an increase in the number of gout cases was most to be feared. If anyone was threatened by pellagra, it was just the "loafing crowd."[23]

The Public Health Service and President Harding were unmoved by the avalanche of denials. While the public outcry was great, many people in the South, including country doctors, agricultural workers, and tenant farmers, wrote either the White House or the PHS to say that food was indeed scarce.

A Mississippi attorney testified that the price of lean meat had risen so high that it was out of the reach of the poor. A Georgia lumberman said that a person must take with a grain of salt what the papers and the health board said about there being no pellagra and plenty to eat. A rural teacher in Arkansas wrote to the President that the better class of people denied conditions of poverty because they had not been out into the country to see the true situation. Times were just as hard as the President had said. The Charity (State) Hospital in Vicksburg, Mississippi, refused admission to pellagra patients because it had no room for them. The insane were sent either to the asylum or to jail—the jail more often than not since the asylum was so crowded with pellagra patients that summer. In Memphis, too, the Pellegra Hospital was full, and patients were turned away.[24]

The better class of people know pellagra exists and is generally connected with poverty, an Alabama agriculture agent wrote the President, but it so reflects on their economic status and general intelligence they want to suppress widespread public attention to an "unfortunate condition of long duration." Wealthier Southerners could truthfully state they had never seen a case. They did not want to see one. Only when a great war submitted the sons of these people to physical examination was it obvious that the pattern of life was destructive of physical health. There were a few newspaper editors in the South who warned against resentment and sensitivity and urged Southerners to act constructively, welcome the aid of the PHS, and educate the people.[25]

Some Southerners denounced the one-crop system. "Why should we pose as 'plumed knights' when we are nothing more nor less than serfs clothing the world below cost to us," wrote one in a letter to the editor of *The State*. Others agreed that for a man to put all his dependence on cotton was not only bad economics but bad psychology as well. When prices were good for cotton the poor farmers of both races tended to take things easy. They quit cultivating their gardens or raising chickens and did nothing but look after the cotton crop. Then, when the price dropped, as it did every seven to ten years, the tenant farmers were out of the habit of working a garden or supplying themselves with food. What the South most needed, an official of a Texas charity organization pointed out, was not a handout of money or food, but education for poor farmers. *The Greensboro Daily News* put it more succinctly: "We need a new system of agriculture."[26]

The impetus for such a new system was at hand. The boll weevil invaded Texas about 1892 and made its way steadily across the South, reaching Georgia by 1916 and South Carolina the following year. The year of the great furor over pellagra was also the year the weevil triumphed. It destroyed more than a third of the cotton crop. Damage was so bad in South Carolina, the editor of *The Spartanburg Journal* observed that "it would have been the wisest and safest thing had not a single bale of cotton been produced in the South."[27] Dr. Wheeler, who remained in the Spartanburg field office of the PHS throughout the summer of 1921, took advantage of this obvious opportunity to drive home a few points about the necessity for a diversified agriculture. The boll weevil might prove the end of pellagra, he told the local Kiwanis Club. If the weevil made the South produce more cattle, sheep, and hogs, more fruit and vegetables, more butter and eggs, and more grain, then the diet of the South would be changed and pellagra would be checked.[28]

"Next year, next year," went the refrain, the agriculture of the South was going to be changed. In 1919 the people of Enterprise, Alabama, had erected a monument to the boll weevil in appreciation to that insect as "the herald of prosperity." Other groups, from bankers to automobile dealers, also preached the necessity of diversified farming. But Georgia's Congressman Wright, in protesting that "cotton will once more be enthroned as king," was more nearly attuned to the Southern mind than those who talked of diversification. Southerners persisted in trying to prop cotton back on the throne, and diversification was more a dream than a reality. "A perennial Southern growth," George B. Tindall has called the diversification campaign. But the growth did not flourish. "The routines of tenancy yielded with difficulty to other arrangements; the marketing, supply, and credit systems were geared to staple crops."[29]

The new excitement over pellagra, after a period of relative quiescence, pumped new life into the peddlers of patent medicine. A dozen or more wrote both the President and the Public Health Service offering to sell their cures for the "benefit" of mankind. Newspaper advertisements of pellagra cures already on the market also appeared. The mails brought more interesting suggestions to the Surgeon General's office than quack remedies, however. A processor of nuts wrote to suggest that peanuts, either cooked or raw, would go far toward offering relief to pellagrins, and at least two laboratories offered to supply yeast to pellagra victims. The offer was refused.[30] Had it been accepted, the work on pellagra would have taken giant strides ahead. Several years later brewer's yeast was found to be the richest source of the pellagra-preventive substance. The lowly peanut, too, came into its own as a valuable food in preventing and curing pellagra.

The Public Health Service was much more interested in the offer of the Institute of American Meat Packers to donate 20,000 pounds of meat for distribution in the South, and of the Borden Milk Company to furnish without charge condensed milk for use in combating the disease. The fierce pride of the South prevented the acceptance of either of these offers. The Southern Commercial Congress even scheduled a conference on pellagra so that an organized effort could be made to bring relief to the stricken farmers and tenants, but the conference was cancelled after state reports minimized the pellagra danger. The South refused charity and advice from whatever quarter it was offered.[31]

Goldberger had wanted to call a meeting of state health officers, agricultural experts, and relief agencies to devise an aid program for pellagra victims in 1921 and to plan for 1922. Such a conference was called for August 4–5 in Washington, but it proved to be something less than the constructive session Goldberger envisioned. Instead, it was a forum in which irate Southern health officials vented their anger against Goldberger and everybody else who dared to "slander" the South. The health officers from the Southern states met behind closed doors in Washington with Goldberger, Surgeon General Cumming and others from the Public Health Service, representatives of the U.S. Department of Agriculture, and Red Cross officials.

Goldberger opened the conference with an explanation of why he had said there were 100,000 cases of pellagra in the South that year. It was not a number he had pulled out of thin air, but rather one at which he had arrived after the most careful consideration. Pellagra was a reportable disease in only one-third of the Southern states. In the other two-thirds, he had to estimate the number of cases as best he could from census death reports and from observation. For his hotly disputed estimate that year, he had relied on the trend of incidence in three localities: the state of Mississippi, Spartanburg County, South Carolina, and the Georgia State Sanitarium. In Mississippi, the number of cases was double in the first six months of 1921 what it had been the year before. In the Inman Mills village in South Carolina, where a house-to-house survey was made, there were more than twice as many cases as in 1920; and at the Georgia State Sanitarium almost 50 percent more pellagra cases had been admitted that year. Goldberger thought it reasonable to assume from these figures that there was a probable increase over 1920 of at least 50 percent, but to be conservative, he reduced this by half. With 80,000 cases in 1920, he estimated 100,000, for 1921. He denied he ever said there would be 10,000 pellagra deaths, as the newspapers had reported. He predicted 5,000 deaths, or about 5 percent of the total number of cases.[32]

No explanation satisfied the angry health officers present, and none was angrier than Goldberger's old adversary, Hayne. He was more explosive at the Washington conference than he had been six years earlier when results of the prison experiment were announced. He vowed that he had not accepted the diet theory of pellagra, that, indeed, he did not expect to accept it, and that he was "not the only fool in South Carolina" who had not accepted it. In a poll he took of South Carolina doctors on whether they subscribed to Goldberger's theory, there were more who said "no" than "yes." His composure failed him completely when he discussed the famine charge. He called it a lie. Equally upset was Alabama's Dr. Samuel W. Welch. The flamboyant newspaper articles "disturbed his poise" and the offer of free meat to Alabamans was such a provocation he could not control himself. Welch insisted the danger of a pellagra increase in Alabama was slight, although he did not try to prove it with figures: "I have never had to verify my statements with letters and figures, as some of my neighbors do."[33]

Vehement denials of any pellagra increase also came from the health officers of Florida and Tennessee, both of whom generously extended invitations to unbelievers to visit their states and behold the bounty. From Mississippi, however, there was an admission that there was a distinct pellagra problem and that Goldberger perhaps was conservative in his estimates. Mississippi's health officer, Leathers, with obvious disregard of the statement he had made but a week earlier in which he branded as ridiculous reports of a pellagra epidemic, refused to "mince matters" with the people of Mississippi. There was a pellagra problem, and Leathers wanted them to know about it. Arkansas, too, admitted that the disease had increased in that state.[34]

There was a dilemma at the conference that was not readily resolved. It was highly unusual for a President to show interest in public health matters, and there was a natural tendency to want to take advantage of President Harding's concern. At the same time, his interest appeared in the unpleasant guise of an insult to the South, and the health officers felt an obligation to defend the honor of the homeland. At the Washington conference, these health officers were public officials first and doctors second. Southern public officials, almost as one, had denounced the "famine and plague" charge, and health officers had followed suit. With pellagra such a hot political issue, they probably were afraid to admit publicly the Public Health Service was right. Surgeon General Cumming used all the skill he could muster to keep the conference from attributing sectional prejudice to the President's remarks. It was a difficult task. The charge of famine and plague had stirred the blood, and Southern pride was strong. The health officers applauded when one of them stated emphatically that Southerners did not appreciate the way in which President Harding had singled out the South as the only part of the country having economic conditions bordering on famine. The South had been injured, and the South was resentful. But in the end, the Surgeon General and reason prevailed. The "tremendous asset" of the President's interest in the health of the people of the United States was too choice a plum to throw away. Kentucky's health director, Dr. A. T. McCormick, urged other health officers to take advantage of this boost from the White House. He put it succinctly: fight the disease, not the President. The state health officials did not request a White House conference on health, as the Public Health Service wished them to do, but at least they refrained from attacking President Harding's motives directly. Instead, they attributed his famine and plague charge to a misinterpretation of terms.[35]

There were a few moments at the conference when passionate oratory gave way to a calm presentation of facts. Such was the case when Dr. Clyde King, an economist employed by the congressional Joint Commission on Agriculture, described the financial depression that had struck so hard at the farmers of the United States, especially farm laborers and tenants. The purchasing power of the farmers' dollar was substantially lower in 1921 than it had been at any other period since 1890. The lowest point previously reached was in 1896 when, as in May 1921, it was 77, a drop from an average of 110 in 1919. For cotton farmers, the situation was more desperate. The purchasing power of their dollar stood at only 66 in May 1921. Such a depression, King said, inevitably caused an increase in disease.[36]

Purchasing power reduced, cotton farmers were further hurt because they had no food resources of their own to fall back on. A USDA farm economist testified that there were few gardens in the plantation districts. Most planters did not have them for their own use, and not more than 10 percent of laborers had gardens. More often than not, these were planted too late to amount to anything. The problem was not only one of few gardens, but also of warped tastes. Some people would not eat good food when it was available, but preferred corn bread and bacon. Repeatedly the need for education on diet was cited. People had to be taught that good food was vital. The problem of milk production and consumption was especially acute. Some tenant farmers, Negroes especially, would not milk a cow or care for a cow, and, if they had the money to buy food, they would not spend it for milk, which was quite expensive.[37]

It was the unavailability of the right kind of food that was the basic problem in pellagra, not poverty per se. PHS statistician Edgar Sydenstricker testified that there were many more poor people in the North and East than in the South, but in those two sections the supply of pellagra-preventing food was available to all; in the South, it was available only to those with relatively high incomes. The trend toward diversification of farm products in the South was not yet great enough to affect the availability of the right kinds of food to mill workers and tenant farmers. Unless some marked changes were made in the availability of food supplies, Sydenstricker thought the outlook not favorable for 1922. He did not believe that the disease would reach the heights it had in 1915, but it was almost certain to be worse in 1922 than it had been in 1920 or even 1921.[38]

The state health officers were in no mood to plan for the rainy day they did not believe was coming. They had come to Washington primarily to protest the slanderous charges against the South, and they concentrated on this. A committee of five was appointed to draw up the resolutions.[39] One member of the committee predicted quite accurately in advance that the report that came out of the conference would not amount to much, that it would simply admit that there was pellagra, that everybody was working on it, and that there was no famine in the South. The resolutions, in fact, skipped lightly over the first two of these points and concentrated on the last. State health officers of the Southern states "deplore the fact that an impression has been created that famine conditions exist in the South," the resolutions began. This was not strong enough for

Dr. Olin West of Tennessee, who unsuccessfully tried to change the word "deplore" to "resent." He and other hard-line officers lost another round, too, when, after brisk discussion, the sentence stating that the pellagra situation was in "no sense more serious than during the past several years" was deleted. The resolutions admitted an increase in some localities, but said there was no cause for alarm. The only plans for the future which the state health officers approved was one calling vaguely for "sane educational methods" and more financial support for federal, state, and local health departments. The honor of the South was salvaged, and the good news was trumpeted throughout the land. *The Atlanta Constitution,* for instance, used a seven-column headline to declare that the pellagra–famine charge had been branded false.[40]

In his official report of the conference to the President, Surgeon General Cumming blamed much of the South's anger over the famine charge to a misinterpretation of the word. As used by the Public Health Service, famine implied a deficiency in certain elements in the diet, but that was not the way it was generally interpreted in the South. People there defined famine in the general rather than the technical sense. To them it meant a severe shortage of all food. In spite of the furor, or perhaps because of it, the Surgeon General was grateful for the President's letter. He thought it was "fortunate" because it made evident the necessity for a concentrated attack on all problems related to public health. Such an attack, he wrote, could best be carried out if all federal agencies concerned with public welfare were brought together in one department. Then federal activities could be coordinated more easily with those of state and local welfare agencies. The creation of a department of welfare was thereafter one of the things to which President Harding gave his strongest support.[41]

Some Southerners had almost as much trouble comprehending Cumming's new definition of "famine" as they had in understanding President Harding's use of the word in the first place.

A "Scientific Famine?" *The Spartanburg Herald* asked. "Surgeon General Cumming has not coined a word, but he has certainly coined a new kind of famine. We have never had a scientific famine in this country before." The people of Spartanburg were perhaps more sensitive than most other Southerners to the "famine" charge because much of the information on which Goldberger's report was based came from the mill villages of the county. The local press tried to rescue the reputation of the region from the aspersions cast upon it. Spartanburg was singled out because for years it had cooperated with health officials when other communities had refused to do so. The Spartanburg County Medical Society had welcomed first the Thompson–McFadden Commission and later representatives from the Public Health Service. Because it served as a base for the most conspicuous authorities on pellagra, the rumor got around that Spartanburg was the center of the trouble. "To be misrepresented is one of the penalties of unselfish service," *The Herald* editor wrote.[42]

It seemed there was no end to the injuries heaped upon Spartanburg for her cooperation. In late August came a three-cents-a-pound offer from a Boston firm for Spartanburg's low-grade spinnable cotton. The insulting offer was attributed to reports of famine in the section and to the belief generated by these reports that South Carolina farmers were starving.[43]

Despite fervent denials that there was an increase in pellagra in the South in 1921, the number of cases did rise that year. In Inman Mills, South Carolina, the village where Goldberger did his intensive survey, there was an increase of approximately 150 percent over 1920. In rural Mississippi, the number of deaths from pellagra in 1921 was 783; in 1920, it had been 558. In South Carolina as a whole, there was a definite rise, which not even Hayne could deny. The annual report of the South Carolina State Board of Health in 1921 showed that the death rate from pellagra for every 100,000 people in the population was 18.5, an increase of about 20 percent from the 15.6 of the year before. This was almost exactly the rate Goldberger had predicted and that Hayne so hotly had denied. In all, there were 2,541 pellagra deaths in the United States that year, but the census registration area did not include Alabama, Georgia, Arkansas, and Texas, states in which the disease was known to be prevalent.[44]

The satisfaction of being proved right, of having his worst fears confirmed, was not what Goldberger wanted. He had hoped to stimulate a cooperative program between federal and state health agencies, which would keep pellagra from spreading so rapidly in the wake of depressed cotton prices. Instead, his warning had only created a tempest which did nothing to protect the South's health. In the end, only Mississippi took the warning seriously and asked for help. Ten days after the Washington conference, George Wheeler was on his way to Mississippi to survey the situation and make recommendations.

What he saw there quickly convinced him that the task ahead was going to be difficult. In the rich delta region, he found a paradox. The finest cotton-growing section of the world had given birth to a way of life that kept most of the people poor and many of them sick. With one-fifth of the state's population, the delta had three-fifths of Mississippi's pellagra cases. Wheeler found that the diet of the delta—the standard meat, meal, and molasses—came about in the most natural way. It was imperishable and highly suited to the commissary, and, just as important, it was easily prepared, palatable, filling, and cheap. Tenants seemed uninterested in keeping cows or growing a garden. Wheeler predicted the job of reform would be difficult. To persuade people to grow food first, and cotton second, was a job that the agricultural agencies, backed by the Southern press, had been unable to accomplish after some years of effort.[45]

He suggested two lines of action. First, essential foods had to be made more available, and second, people had to be educated to eat them. In upland Mississippi, where the boll weevil had already driven farmers to a more diversified agriculture, it was enough to concentrate on the second step. In the delta, however, the first problem was to get the right kind of food to the people. Wheeler suggested that Mississippi health officials send to the region a person who was trained in public health and who understood the delta's peculiar agricultural and economic conditions. When visiting planters and tenants, this health official could work for a better diet, not by disparaging the use of the three-M's, but by encouraging the use of some good pellagra-preventing supplements. Like Goldberger, Wheeler thought the key to the whole problem was increased consumption of milk.[46]

While Wheeler was in Mississippi trying to work out a program for a state which had admitted at the Washington conference that it was hard-pressed, Florida continued its fight with the government over the famine and plague accusation, the bout which most other states considered they had already won handily. The Florida Development Board, however, was not satisfied. It wanted to know what motive the government had for discriminating against the Southern states. No explanation the PHS offered seemed satisfactory, certainly not the one that it desired only to prevent needless loss of life from one of the most readily preventable diseases. The Florida Development Board continued to insist that the PHS had been careless in preparing the original charge against the South, and a Florida congressman complained that, at every turn, he met some obstacle which intentionally or unintentionally had been placed in the way of further advancement of Florida.[47]

From North Carolina came a blast from health officer Rankin. Countering the PHS report of an increase in pellagra with a report from the Secretary of Agriculture that food supplies were more adequate in the South than usual, he charged the Surgeon General with a "lack of courage" to admit the error in declaring the South in the grip of famine and plague.[48]

This was not the final outburst against Goldberger and his dietary theory. The last volley was fired at the meeting of the Southern Medical Association in Hot Springs, Arkansas, three months after the Washington conference. Dr. Deeks, the nutrition specialist who had gained fame as a member of the Isthmian Canal Commission, was there to defend diet. His own treatment differed from that of Goldberger only in that Deeks stressed the avoidance of carbohydrates. Mississippi's health officer Leathers was also there to speak out for the necessity of a good diet, but these two stood virtually alone. The day belonged to the opposition, and it made the most of it. Infection was the cause of pellagra, they said. Goldberger's prison farm experiment and the transmissibility experiment were dismissed as worthless, and the entire state of Mississippi was held up to ridicule for accepting the Goldberger theory. The high pellagra death rate there was proof enough that something was wrong with the treatment.[49]

Goldberger did not hear these new attacks on his work for he was busy elsewhere; he had gone back to the laboratory. Since 1914 when he began work with pellagra he had found himself on the cutting edge of not one but two new fields of science: nutrition and social medicine. The practicing physicians of the South had rejected his findings in nutrition because they were too deeply schooled in the bacteriological concept of disease to accept them; the politicians, including many of the state health officers, had rejected his efforts to tie pellagra to the basic poverty of the South because they were unwilling to admit that the South was poor. As a public relations man, Goldberger was a failure. He did his work in virtual seclusion and then sprang what appeared to be startling findings on an unprepared public. As a social reformer—for that was what he was that summer of 1921 even though he probably did not look at it that way—he was hardly a success. He succeeded in making people angry, but he did not change the Southern system of agriculture. As a medical detective, however, he was a genius. Before his critics gathered in Hot Springs, he was deeply involved in a new task, a systematic search for the nutritive ingredient that was missing from the meat, meal, and molasses diet of the South.

7

The Quiet
Search

THE HUBBUB OF THE SUMMER of 1921 marked the halfway
point in Goldberger's fifteen-year study of pellagra. That summer, even as the Washington conference was underway, his own
work took a new turn. The search for "something missing" in
the pellagrin's diet was work for the hand to do, less dramatic
than curing hundreds of orphans with a good diet or inducing
pellagra in a group of prisoners with a poor one, but essential
work nonetheless. What Goldberger had proved in the field,
he had now to prove in the laboratory. Compared to the years
that went before, this was a quiet time. Whereas he once spent
weeks on the road visiting cities from Virginia and the Carolinas
to Texas, in the 1920s he reduced his field of operations to
two points: the Hygienic Laboratory in Washington and the
Georgia State Sanitarium at Milledgeville. It was from Milledgeville that he wrote home some good news in late September
1921: "We have found a road which . . . will come close to
nailing pellagra's old hide to the barn door."[1]

The road was one he had selected four years before, not knowing quite where it would lead. In 1917, Dr. W. F. Tanner,

a new associate, set to work systematically testing one item of food after another for its effectiveness in preventing pellagra. Goldberger hoped he would find something that was both cheap and readily available. It was not enough to recommend to poor people that they eat fresh meat and eggs and drink milk when they lacked both the money to buy these foods and the inclination to provide them for themselves. He needed a cheap substitute. The search for one was conducted at the Georgia State Sanitarium where conditions were easily controlled and material for observation abundant.[2]

Their work began logically enough with beans. Goldberger and Tanner began testing soybeans and peas in 1917—soybeans because they were high in food value, cheap, and handy, and blackeyed peas, or cowpeas, because they were a staple in many Southern diets. For months, hundreds of women patients were given a monotonous but hopefully pellagra-preventive diet consisting largely of soybeans or peas. To Goldberger's disappointment, his faith in the miracle value of beans was not sustained. What his statistical studies in South Carolina had shown was confirmed in this practical test: beans would not prevent pellagra.[3]

Systematically, the search for the missing quantity in the pellagrin's diet was narrowed. It was known that proteins, mineral salts, and three vitamins—fat-soluble A, antineuritic B, and scurvy-preventing C—were necessary for health. Diets designed to test the efficacy of each of these elements were developed. Mineral supplements were checked first. A group of patients considered liable to the disease was given mixtures of mineral salts containing all the inorganic elements of a liter of whole milk, an amount known to prevent pellagra. These salts, mixed with the breakfast cereal, or hash or into some part of the midday meal, were ineffective. The known vitamins, A, B, and C, were also ruled out. The regular diet at the sanitarium contained at least a minimum amount of these vitamins for there were few signs of eye disorders, beriberi, or scurvy there.[4]

The proteins were still to be tested. In the summer of 1921, while tempers flared throughout the South over accusations of famine and plague, testing of the protein supply at Milledgeville began. Goldberger and Tanner started with gelatin and made plans to work later with other kinds of protein, including beef and casein. Goldberger correctly predicted that gelatin would prove of no value, but he expected good results from beef and casein. These studies were preliminary to a systematic investigation of the therapeutic value of certain amino acids, which he anticipated would aid eventually in finding the cause of pellagra.[5]

Proteins are composites of amino acids, sixteen of which had been found by 1900. At least one of these, tryptophan, absent in the digestion of corn or maize, was known to be essential for survival. It was the initial success with tryptophan that so stirred Goldberger's hopes in the early fall of 1921 that he thought he was on the way toward "nailing pellagra's hide to the barn door."

On August 1, 1921, while Goldberger was busy in Washington preparing for the conference of state health officers, Tanner in Milledgeville began to give a half-dram of tryptophan before each meal to a seriously ill pellagra victim. The patient showed immediate improvement. Three days later his skin looked better, and by the next day he was markedly improved. On August 5, the very day the state health officers concluded their stormy session and left Washington for their homes amidst a blaze of publicity, Tanner wrote Goldberger the condition of the patient was nearly normal, the erythema almost entirely gone, and the blebs healed without bursting. Tanner commented, "the improvement in this patient's skin condition has surpassed anything I have ever seen in a case of pellagra in an equal period of time."[6] It was ironic that the important news about pellagra that August 5 came not from angry Southerners but in a quiet personal letter to the man who had been the object of so much wrath.

The work with amino acids was conducted on a very small scale because amino acids were expensive. Goldberger wanted to test three of them—tryptophan, cystine, and lysine—and in the autumn of 1920 had requested a $1,000 appropriation to underwrite a study which he admitted would be so small that it could at best afford only suggestive indications. The initial results were so dramatic, however, that a year later he asked for another $12,500 so that tests on a scale large enough to be conclusive could be conducted. He thought this would be enough to feed ten people for six months, long enough to give conclusive results, narrowing the question of an amino acid deficiency to very restricted limits.[7]

Such a deficiency would answer many questions about pellagra. It would explain why people of the Central Powers in Europe, who had suffered from severe malnutrition during and after the war, did not have pellagra. Whatever the dietary deficiency that caused the disease, it was not missing from the diets of these people. It would also explain why pellagra occasionally occurred in nursing infants, a point often used to refute the dietary theory. These children were not getting enough biologically good protein to meet their needs. On the basis of practical experience, Goldberger suggested that diets should contain a minimum of forty grams of animal protein a day.

While Goldberger and Tanner seemed confident they were on the right track, they did not rule out the possibility that some yet unknown dietary factor might be involved. Within a few months they were to change the course of their search and join the ranks of the vitamin hunters themselves, but they were perfectly correct in attributing pellagra to an amino acid deficiency. Time was to reveal a peculiar relationship between tryptophan and the pellagra-preventing vitamin.[8]

In his experiments at Milledgeville, Goldberger built on the work of others, especially chemists and animal husbandrymen, who were slowly molding a new way of thinking about food. It had been but twenty years since public interest in food centered on the calorie. Then from England in 1906 came the discovery of Hopkin's "accessory food factors," something essential to life but not revealed by any known analytical methods. Gradually the scientific world accepted these new facts of life, and even more gradually laymen learned that they could not live by bread alone, certainly not the kind of bread the South doted on. To try to do so was to "starve."[9]

Chemical analysis had been used from about 1860 to the early years of the twentieth century to determine the amount of nutrients in food. Devised in Germany, this method was universally accepted by agricultural chemists to determine quickly the values of various feedstuffs. The only essentials believed to be necessary were proteins, plus carbohydrates and fats for energy, and a few mineral salts. When supplied in sufficient quantity, from whatever source, these elements would insure growth and health and the production of milk, meat, eggs, and wool. The first to question the infallibility of this system was Stephen M. Babcock, a New York-born farmboy who went to Germany in the late 1870s to learn what the giants of chemistry were teaching there. He learned the accepted methods of analyzing foods, the practical object being to select the most economical diet possible for farm animals. But there was a flicker of doubt in his mind, even as a student in Germany, that chemical analysis of foods told everything there was to know. He had not been back in the United States long before he was sure it did not. Working with healthy, well-fed cows at the Experiment Station at Geneva, New York, he learned that if he ignored the mineral content of the cows' food, by chemical analysis they excreted exactly the same amount of proteins, carbohydrates, and fats they had eaten. Since cows had to assimilate much of what they eat and since nothing was wrong with them, something had to be wrong with the analysis.

By 1890, a couple of years after Babcock moved to the College of Agriculture at the University of Wisconsin, chemists and animal husbandrymen had lost faith in the German system of chem-

---

ical analysis in planning farm rations. Babcock, a man of great good humor, told W. O. Atwater, America's outstanding authority on human nutrition in the 1890s and the man who devised the means of measuring food energy in calories, that according to chemical analysis soft coal would be as good a food for pigs as farm crops, and a great deal cheaper. Soft coal contained nitrogen, which made up 16 percent of most proteins. Multiply the nitrogen content of a food by 6.25 and the protein content could be known. Soft coal also contained ether-soluble substances, which food analysis called fat. Carbohydrates or energy were supplied by other fractions. According to chemical analysis, soft coal was a splendid food. The humorless Atwood did not appreciate the analogy.

One of the most famous experiments to determine the value of particular foods for farm animals was begun by Babcock at Wisconsin in 1907. Working with a young chemist, E. B. Hart, and the new professor of animal husbandry, G. C. Humphrey, he began to feed cows from a single-plant source: one group on maize, one on oats, one on wheat. The parts of the plants were combined so that the rations would have a similar chemical analysis. If the progress of all groups was the same, then the chemical data must be accepted as reliable. If there was a difference, it would show that there were some factors in food not yet detectable by chemical methods. In time the cows showed distinct differences. Those fed on corn were sleek and gave birth to healthy calves; all the calves born of the oats-fed group died except one; the wheat-fed animals were small, rough-coated, and blind, and their calves were all born dead.

When the experiment was well underway, a young biochemist from Yale University was hired by the Experiment Station to work on the project. "Though all the cows had had feed of the same chemical composition," Elmer V. McCollum wrote years later, "they differed enormously in physiological status. I was employed to discover why this was so. It was a man-sized job for a beginner."[10]

Before Babcock, Hart, Humphrey, and McCollum discovered what was wrong with those cows—that the corn-fed group got leaf and shuck and stalk and the health-giving elements these contained along with the grain, while the oats and wheat-fed groups got just the grain and some straw—McCollum had begun a new kind of work in nutrition, which was to yield much fruit. He began a systematic search for the missing quantity in the diets of rats fed on purified proteins, carbohydrates, fats, and inorganic salts. Working with his rat colony, he discovered vitamin A, and he initiated a new way of testing the nutritional value of foods through biological analysis: he fed his rats certain purified diets, then added one item at a time and watched for results.

This was the technique Goldberger used at Milledgeville. Giving patients the hospital's standard starchy diet, he added one item at a time and watched. Small-scale tests proved the effectiveness of fresh beef and buttermilk (more popular in the rural South than fresh milk) in preventing pellagra, and the ineffectiveness of gelatin, butter, and cod-liver oil.[11] The butter was used to test for McCollum's vitamin A and the cod-liver oil for McCollum's vitamin D, discovered at Johns Hopkins University in 1922.

While overseeing the practical work at Milledgeville, Goldberger spent much of his time in Washington where the technical work on pellagra was done. The Hygienic Laboratory was a busy place in these years, headquarters for research and study on many different diseases, including some of the most virulent infections known to man. Goldberger's work in nutrition was just one of many problems with which the laboratory dealt. Its long-time concern with diphtheria, rabies, and smallpox control continued, and the staff began work on allergies—unraveling the mysteries of serum shock—and initiated investigations of diseases like tularemia, poliomyelitis, Rocky Mountain spotted fever, brucellosis, and psittacosis. During the 1920s, the laboratory developed a vaccine for spotted fever, confirmed the similarity of human and cattle strains of brucellosis, and found that psittacosis, or parrot fever, was caused by a filterable virus, diffused through the air like pollen. Although Goldberger worked in several areas of research during these years, including investigations of typhus fever, his main concern was pellagra. In 1922 when the laboratory's Division of Pathology was divided into three sections, he was appointed chief of the section on nutritional diseases.[12]

That same year Goldberger found that dogs could be used as experimental animals for pellagra study, so for the first time since 1914 when PHS officer Edward Francis tried unsuccessfully to give rhesus monkeys pellagra by feeding them hominy grits, rutabaga turnips, kale, and syrup, work with animals began. Goldberger had toyed with the idea of working with dogs since 1915 when he read in Russell H. Chittenden's *The Nutrition of Man* that dogs, when switched from a diet of meat and milk to one containing mostly bread, showed a dramatic change for the worse in as little as four days, and in fact, seemed to suffer from something similar to human pellagra. Goldberger had tried twice without success to duplicate Chittenden's experiment, but in early 1922 he decided to try once more.[13]

His first problem was to determine the nature of the pellagra-like syndrome which Chittenden had observed. It was not long before he strongly suspected that it was black tongue, known to veterinarians throughout the South and generally regarded as infectious. The disease seemed to come on suddenly with lassitude and loss of appetite. More violent symptoms quickly followed—a sore mouth, some vomiting, and diarrhea. In little more than a week, 75 percent of the animals died. A Texan noted that in a strip of his state where there was a great deal of pellagra, the people could not keep dogs because they died of sore mouth. Goldberger observed that black tongue and pellagra had the same geographic distribution. As soon as he was able definitely to produce a pellagralike disease in dogs through faulty feeding and have the diagnosis confirmed as black tongue, he was ready to begin his experimental work on a larger scale. Black tongue and pellagra were essentially the same disease.[14] Having at last found a suitable experimental animal, the pellagra work accelerated.

When Goldberger began his full-scale work with dogs in January 1922, the standard diet he gave them consisted of grits, wheat farina, rice, cowpeas, milk, lard, gelatin, cod-liver oil, and tomato juice. To stimulate their appetites and build them up for the tests ahead, he added one cake of commercial yeast to each daily ration. Six months later, the animals were not eating well, so the amount of yeast was doubled. By November 1922, the dogs showed some signs of mange but none of black tongue. Although he did not recognize it at once, Goldberger had found in yeast the richest source of the pellagra-preventive substance.

Early in 1923 Goldberger and Wheeler reorganized their work with dogs. They began to feed groups of dogs on the most potent pellagra-producing diet they could conceive. The diet they had used in 1922 contained some milk because the diets of pellagra victims often contained a little milk and a small amount of meat. In 1923 they eliminated milk altogether, substituted cottonseed oil for part of the cod-liver oil, and eliminated the yeast since it did not ordinarily enter into the diet of people with pellagra, even in their bread. Even then they did not suspect that yeast possessed the much sought after pellagra preventive. As signs of black tongue appeared, the doctors modified the diets adding a single new foodstuff. They first tested meat; later they added other foods one at a time. If the dog got well, that food was added to the list of pellagra-preventives. If the dog died, that food was dropped from consideration.[15]

That year they tested soybeans and found that in small amounts they were ineffective in preventing black tongue. When given in very large amounts (360 grams daily), they proved fairly effective. Soybeans contained some pellagra-preventive factor, but not very much. They tested skim milk, and found that it, too, was effective if consumed in large enough quantity. Carrots, rutabagas, butter, cod-liver oil, cottonseed oil, egg yolk, and whole corn were ruled out as pellagra preventives. The best results were with lean beef, pork liver, salmon, wheat germ, and yeast. Results with yeast were almost magical. Within four days after a dog with black tongue was given yeast, there was marked improvement. If yeast were taken away, black tongue reappeared. At the laboratory they could make the disease appear and disappear at will. In this respect, its mystery of two hundred years was stripped away. The work progressed, as Goldberger expressed it, with "unanticipated speed."[16]

Meanwhile, at Milledgeville, Tanner duplicated experiments in the Washington laboratory, testing one food after another. He tried butter with one group, cod-liver oil with another, purified casein with a third, and finally supplemental minerals and vitamin-rich foods with a fourth group. Butter and cod-liver oil were ineffective even though given in massive amounts—five ounces of butter or four-and-a-half ounces of cod-liver oil a day. Casein, on the other hand, proved quite effective in preventing dermatitis, although it did not prevent the recurrence of some other symptoms of the disease.[17]

It was with yeast, however, that Goldberger and Tanner got their most dramatic results. On May 26, 1923, two patients at Milledgeville were given yeast for the first time. Results were so favorable that the experiment was expanded during the next year until there were twenty-six patients taking dried brewer's yeast daily, most often mixed in with the syrup served at supper. All the patients showed improvement in two to three days. Results with yeast were so convincing that the theory of an amino acid deficiency had to be discarded. Yeast contained too little protein for this theory to be supported. Goldberger coined a new name for the potent health-giving ingredient of yeast. He called it the pellagra-preventive factor, or for short, factor P-P.[18]

Yeast had much to recommend it. Not only was it effective in preventing pellagra, but it did not spoil readily and it was cheap. Goldberger and Tanner tried brewer's yeast and bakers' yeast. Both worked, but it took a much larger quantity of the latter to effect a cure. The good results achieved with yeast were reported in two articles in *Public Health Reports* in 1925. The public press, too, announced that yeast would cure pellagra. For many people the word came not a day too soon. It was spring, and pellagra was making its annual appearance throughout the South. Some victims of the disease who did not know where to get the almost magical yeast wrote Goldberger begging him to send it to them COD.[19]

Goldberger was meticulous. He was not satisfied to find one good, inexpensive source of factor P-P. He still hoped to find it in foods that Southerners might easily eat every day. He worked with dry skim milk beginning the summer of 1923 but found that it was not a particularly rich source. Dissatisfied with his early experiments with beef when only eight patients were included, Goldberger conducted the experiment on a larger scale during 1924 and 1925. There were twenty-six patients in this test, who received almost seven ounces of ground beef a day, equally divided between lunch and dinner. None of the patients developed pellagra, but five developed symptoms of beriberi, which cleared up when they were given more whole cornmeal and cowpeas. He tested butter again, thinking that perhaps the Georgia-produced butter, which he had used in the first test, was inferior because the Georgia pastures were poor. In the second experiment, he used butter from Vermont, but it proved no more effective in preventing pellagra.[20]

All the tests with food lasted for at least a year, and, during that time, the mentally ill women, mostly Negroes, who participated in them ate the same food day after day. The basic diet was cornmeal, served either as corn bread or mush, cowpeas, wheat flour, lard, and a small serving of tomato juice. To this was added one other item: butter or beef or skim milk or something else. One group got large glasses of tomato juice (far above the amount in the regular diet) three times a day. Another had a pound of carrots allotted to each patient daily. The carrots were steamed and mashed and stirred into other foods at lunch and supper. A third group ate rutabagas, a pound a day for each patient. A little later, the test groups at Milledgeville were given wheat germ, which was boiled with the other cereals in the diet. In 1927 they tested canned salmon. Using a group of white women, the PHS officers fed each patient six ounces of salmon a day, mixed with grits or mush. From this series of monotonous diets came some valuable information. Tomatoes were found to prevent pellagra completely if as much as forty ounces a day were used. A pound of carrots or rutabagas a day was not enough to prevent pellagra, but Goldberger suggested that more might work. Wheat germ was so effective that he proposed that some of the milling products of the wheat be added to flour in the pellagra areas. Salmon, too, worked well. This was important to know because canned salmon was popular in the South, and it was comparatively cheap.[21]

Even before results of the diet tests at Milledgeville were announced to the public, officials at the Georgia State Sanitarium were praising the Public Health Service. In 1915, there were 210 patients at the hospital with a psychosis due to pellagra; in 1925, there were but 23. Goldberger and Wheeler, who had replaced Tanner at the hospital in 1924, "robbed the disease of much of its mystery and many of its terrors," the sanitarium superintendent noted in his annual report. A few years later, hospital officials observed that the pellagra problem became "more and more simple" as different foods were studied and their values as sources of vitamin P-P made known.[22]

The work of Goldberger and his associates in the 1920s greatly narrowed the scope of the problem, and, although their efforts made it possible for hospital authorities to think of pellagra as "more and more simple," the problem remained complex. The nature of vitamin P-P (or vitamin G, as it was sometimes called) and how it worked was still unknown. In an experiment with white rats, Goldberger and an associate, Dr. R. D. Lillie,

tackled this problem, but its ultimate solution was not known
for another decade. Goldberger thought it probable that a condition analogous to pellagra could be produced in the white rat
by improper feeding. Using a restricted diet, he soon had rats
with erosions around the mouth, ulcerated tongues, and dermatitis affecting the ears and paws. With yeast, he was able to
bring them back from the brink of death. The yeast he used
differed from that he first fed the dogs in Washington and the
patients at Milledgeville in that it had been subjected to heat
under pressure. Autoclaved yeast, unlike that which was un-
heated, did not prevent polyneuritis or permit the animal to
grow even when it composed 40 percent of its diet. If rats were
denied all sources of vitamin B except that in autoclaved yeast,
they sickened and died, but not from pellagra. When supplied
with vitamin B from dried corn, for example, but denied vitamin
P-P from autoclaved yeast, the animals soon developed signs
of pellagra. They thrived only when they received vitamins from
both sources. This evidence suggested to Goldberger what others
had already observed: vitamin B was not a single entity but
consisted of at least two parts. The first was the heat-sensitive
antiberberi vitamin; the second was the heat-stable P-P. It was
conceivable that these two factors were in themselves complexes
containing one or more parts.[23]

During these years of the quiet search, Goldberger's work
was not accepted without question. Hayne of South Carolina,
who had been angry with Goldberger for ten years, ridiculed
the use of yeast, and several more theories on the cause of pellagra were advanced. Physicians in Butler County, Georgia,
meanwhile, continued to list pellagra as a communicable disease.

On the whole, however, these were good years for Goldberger.
The work went well, criticisms of it were minor, and he was
accorded some professional honors. He was elected first a member and then a fellow of the American Association for the Advancement of Science, a fellow of the American Public Health
Association, a member of the Washington Academy of Sciences,

and a member of the Board of Governors of the American College of Physicians.[24]

His greatest achievement came in the wake of a natural disaster. In the spring of 1927 the Mississippi River overflowed its banks in the worst flood of its history. By early June, 112 counties in 12 states were under water, and, weeks after the first levees crumbled, Red Cross workers were still at work. It was not only a problem of rescue, but one of food, clothing, and shelter as well. There was also the problem of health. Malaria and typhoid posed the most immediate threat, so tons of quinine and enough typhoid vaccine for 400,000 people were sent to the flood area. It was not until July that a third serious threat to health appeared. This was pellagra, which had a habit of coming on the heels of disaster and hard times. Because of the flood, food was scarcer than usual, and pellagra, which had been sharply on the increase for several years, jumped to new heights. Health officers did what they always did when pellagra reared its head high enough for the public to see. They sent for Goldberger. In late July he left with Edgar Sydenstricker for a tour of the flood area in Tennesseee, Mississippi, Arkansas, and Louisiana. Goldberger's description of what he saw there moved his wife to tears; his report on what needed to be done moved the Red Cross to a new kind of action.[25]

The flood area offered a giant testing ground for the new theory of vitamins versus pellagra. Based on a house-to-house survey of Sunflower County, Mississippi, where 102 cases of pellagra appeared among a population of 4,100, Goldberger and Sydenstricker estimated that there would be 45,000 to 50,000 cases in the 4 states they visited. The remedy they proposed for the immediate relief of the giant misery was brewer's yeast, tons of it for thousands of victims. In the next few months, the Red Cross distributed 12,000 pounds of it. This was the first time powdered yeast was used as a public health measure.[26]

The recommended "dose" of yeast was two teaspoonfuls three times a day for adults, or half that much for children. The majority of cases were cured within six to ten weeks, and the cost was but three cents a day. Because it was unpalatable, yeast was often mixed with milk or molasses or fruit juice to disguise the flavor. In whatever way it was given, it worked. Pellagrins, given but ten days to live, got well.[27] That year Goldberger's months of work with dogs in his Washington laboratory and with the insane women at Milledgeville paid handsome dividends.

In the refugee camps where thousands stayed until the water receded, an educational campaign of a sort was conducted. The food served daily was simple and plain, but it constituted a reasonably balanced diet, something which many were not used to and something which Red Cross officials hoped people would copy when they got home. Yeast, effective as it was, was but a temporary measure. Final solution to the problem lay in a steady proper diet. In refugee camps, only two meals a day were served, but these featured meat, milk, and beans, in addition to the standard grits, bread, and syrup. In the mountains of eastern Kentucky where there also were floods in 1927, a Red Cross nutritionist provided balanced meals in refugee camps for only fifteen cents a day. When people left the camp, they carried food with them. For families in which pellagra was chronic, a special take-home diet was provided. It contained cabbage, canned tomatoes, dried peas, and canned milk in quantity, with salt pork, dried beans, and cornmeal curtailed. Some flood victims received more permanent aid: the gift of a cow. The Red Cross provided cows for many victims; private organizations shipped in cows and other livestock for others. The American Jersey Cattle Club, for example, shipped forty head of cattle to Louisiana to help dairymen there rehabilitate themselves, and the Oregon Buff Orphinton Fanciers Association sent a carload of chickens.[28]

Pellagra did not recede with the flood waters, but rather worsened over the next two years. The delta counties of Mississippi were overrun with pellagrins. In Sharkey and Issaquena counties, 1,200 cases of pellagra were treated in the two years after the flood. As many as 75 pellagrins a day came to the county health office for yeast and food and information on what they could do. In Sunflower County, where pellagra was a serious problem among the plantation tenants, weekly clinics were held at Ruleville and Indianola. The American Legion Auxiliary and the Red Cross furnished yeast to Sunflower residents, and the state board of health distributed it. Health workers persuaded drug and grocery stores in the area to stock brewer's yeast, but none of their efforts to control pellagra were very successful. In Bolivar County, where 1,000 cases of pellagra developed in the two years after the flood in spite of the distribution of hundreds of pounds of yeast, health officials acknowledged that this was hardly a permanent solution. What people really needed were gardens with fresh vegetables and an ample supply of milk.[29]

The real force that kept people from cultivating gardens and drinking fresh milk in the lower Mississippi Valley region was not the flood, although that was the immediate excuse in 1927. It was the peculiar pattern of life that kept so many people in rich farming land undernourished and sick. Goldberger had not said much about the disastrous pattern of agriculture in the South since the debacle of 1921, but after the flood he decided once more to speak his mind. In an article in *Public Health Reports* he blamed pellagra in the South—especially in the plantation region of the Mississippi delta—on the one-crop system of agriculture. He called King Cotton the thief that robbed thousands of their health, keeping vital food crops from being grown and maintaining a stranglehold on the South's economic structure.

Goldberger had gone full circle in the decade since he walked the streets of the mill villages of South Carolina and saw the pitiful poverty there. In 1917 he blamed pellagra on poverty, and he proved it neatly with statistics. In the years between that time and 1927, he worked mostly in the laboratory and found one answer to the pellagra problem in vitamin P-P. The more he saw of devastation in the Mississippi flood area, how-

ever, the more convinced he became that the real cure to pellagra lay not in medicine but in economics. "In the present
situation, the outstanding fact, aside from the deprivation directly due to the recent over-flow," Goldberger wrote in his
report, "is that the economic condition of the entire cotton producing area is unfavorable."[30]

The account that followed was much like what had been
said hundreds of times before and by men better acquainted
with agriculture than he. For a medical man, Goldberger was
plowing relatively new ground. Social medicine was hardly a
new idea, but its roots in America were not very deep. In
tackling the pellagra problem, Goldberger had probably done
as much to advance the field as any other. The task was not
an easy one, but he could agree with the Surgeon General who
a few years earlier had said that research in public health should
not terminate when the purely physical factors of disease had
been determined. Work had to continue until cheap, practicable,
and effective methods of control had been placed at the disposal
of mankind.[31]

Years of work, repeated attacks on his methods and even
his motives, and the discouraging progress made in combating
a disease that he had proved was preventable told on Goldberger.
His hair turned gray; the lines on his face deepened. Paul
De Kruif, bacteriologist and author, visited him at the Hygienic
Laboratory at Christmas time 1927 and again the next June,
the year when pellagra deaths in the United States reached
the highest level since the terrible year of 1915. De Kruif called
him the "soft spoken desperado." Goldberger had done his work
well, but the problem was no nearer solution than ever. He
talked to De Kruif of poverty and human ignorance. As he
turned to go back into the laboratory to work with his dogs
and his rat colony he added. "After all, I'm only a bum doctor,
and what can I do about the economic conditions of the
South?"[32] A long time before, Hayne of South Carolina had
asked Goldberger the same thing.

8

A Practical
Approach

PELLAGRA RESOLVED itself into a question of education and economics. If people could be educated to the true nature of the
disease and its prevention, and if economic conditions could
be improved to obtain an adequate diet, pellagra would disappear. But, as Goldberger had learned, educating people to the
true nature of pellagra was no easy task. Ordinary educational
methods did not suffice among those who lacked the means
to procure an adequate diet. A special approach was also needed
for those who were too ignorant to increase the variety of their
diet even when they had enough money. Cars, tires, and gasoline
often got preference over food. The man who remarked that
pellagra came in the wake of the Model-T Ford was not being
facetious.[1]

The Mississippi River flood jolted many people into an aware-
ness of the social and economic aspects of pellagra, and drought
and depression in the early 1930s brought action. The first evidence of a change in public opinion came at the meeting of
the Southern Medical Association in Memphis in mid-November
1927. The public health section of the association adopted a

resolution recognizing pellagra as a dietary problem "intimately bound up with the economic factors influencing the character of the food supply." Doctors pledged their support to agricultural agencies promoting a diversification of farming and requested every practicing physician in the South to help to make good food more available to farmers and tenants.[2]

The time had come to quit quibbling over the etiology of pellagra. Dr. C. W. Garrison, state health officer of Arkansas, urged doctors instead to throw their energy into preventing the disease, and this meant supporting the agriculturists and their "live at home" programs. When any disease reached the proportions that pellagra had reached in Arkansas (5,000 to 10,000 cases annually, with 500 deaths), it was a problem not just for doctors or economists or statisticians, but for the commonwealth. Arkansas, in fact, turned the problem over to the commonwealth when the governor called a conference of agricultural, educational, health, industrial, commercial, and civic agencies to discuss and promote a long-range program of food production.[3]

Despite this new encouragement from the Southern Medical Association and the state of Arkansas, Goldberger was skeptical about eventual victory over the disease. The incidence of pellagra climbed again in 1928, and, in the last public address of his life, he expressed little hope that pellagra would be conquered soon. Education would help, but genuine improvement could be expected only when there was improvement in basic economic conditions. "This, obviously, cannot be accomplished in a day," he told the American Dietetic Association, "but that day will be hastened by the cooperative action of all whose vision enables them to see the great social and economic advantages to be derived from the eradication of the disease."[4]

Goldberger had a vision of the promised land, but he was not allowed to enter it. He died of cancer in January 1929, a year before pellagra began its decline as some of the measures he had long recommended were at last translated into action.

The eventual success of the program he outlined was a better monument to his work than the tribute heaped upon him by the scientific world at his death. In life, Goldberger never worried much about honors but found his satisfaction within. "I know what I have done," he once told his wife, "and it is a satisfaction to my soul which no one on earth can take from me."[5] In his premature death, he was robbed of the ultimate satisfaction of seeing his life's work bear splendid fruit.

Goldberger died without establishing the exact identity of the pellagra-preventive vitamin, a fact which left plenty of work for others to do and one which gave his critics a new opportunity for attack. His work was vulnerable at this point only because it was incomplete, but this defect was hailed with apparent joy by those who had ideas of their own to put forward. Countering these attacks kept PHS officials from giving full attention to more important matters of pellagra control. At the first meeting of the Southern Medical Association after Goldberger's death, the attack began again. A Jacksonville, Florida, physician launched it with a paper on that old favorite, salvarsan, as a treatment for pellagra. He acknowledged that a good diet was of some value, but he belittled work Goldberger and Wheeler had done in singling out a little known vitamin which "for want of a better name" they called P-P. The work is "inconclusive and we still are almost as much in the dark as in the days when we considered pellagra to be caused in some vague manner by corn." South Carolina's Hayne made another intemperate outburst at the same meeting, one which Wheeler later assured the troubled Mrs. Goldberger did not amount to anything. In open meetings Hayne talked a lot, Wheeler wrote her, but in South Carolina his policies and practices were strictly in accordance with the principles which Goldberger laid down.[6]

Wheeler took up the pellagra investigation on Goldberger's death, and it became his job to defend his mentor's work. The most serious attack on the vitamin theory came from Dr. Sidney Bliss of Tulane University, who said that pellagra was caused by a deficiency of iron, not a deficiency of vitamin P-P, "assuming . . . there is such a 'vitamin.' " Bliss charged in an article in *Science* that Goldberger's work had made less of an impression on clinicians and laboratory workers in the South than might be inferred from its acceptance in the standard texts. He pointed out that foods which were claimed to be rich in vitamin P-P or G were also rich in iron, while molasses and meal, the pellagra-producing foods of the South, were poor in iron. On reading this, Wheeler wrote an indignant letter to the editor of *Science* protesting that Goldberger's work had given clinicians of the South their first and only means by which pellagra could be successfully combated and that his work would endure "so long as facts retain their prestige and significance." But the letter never reached the editor of *Science*. It got no further than the Surgeon General's desk. *JAMA* gave the Bliss iron-deficiency theory a boost a few weeks later when it cited the work in an editorial pointing to the need for vigilance in the face of an increasing prevalence of pellagra as indicated in the figures for 1929. "It has again become 'open season' in the hunt for explanations," *JAMA* commented. The ever-vigilant Wheeler protested to the Surgeon General that the pellagra cause should not be allowed to suffer from such frank misrepresentation of the facts.[7]

There were others who also "misrepresented" the facts, much to the annoyance of the Public Health Service. The infection theory was still being promoted by a few. Dr. Beverley R. Tucker, a Virginia physician, suspected a virus, "a Madam X in the house of death," and called for a complete reinvestigation of the pellagra problem, complete with transmissibility tests on animals and condemned criminals. An exhibit of his work won a prize at the meeting of the Southern Medical Association in 1935. An Egyptian specialist reported success in treating pellagra with daily injections of a common chemical, sodium thiosulphate. He attributed pellagra to a toxin caused by eating beans. The PHS considered such claims "scientifically absurd," not destructive enough to justify experimental refutation, but somewhat dangerous because their publication might hamper the dissemination of useful knowledge.[8]

The gathering and dissemination of such useful knowledge was Wheeler's job. With the enthusiasm of an idealist, he wanted to make the small cotton and tenant farmer of the South "depression proof." He believed the answer lay in local planning, in persuading bankers to take an interest in pellagra control. Bankers, he knew, were taken seriously by cotton farmers. It was far better to get bankers really interested than to depend on the distribution of yeast or the lending of milk cows to wipe out pellagra. Those methods were no more effective than a blow-out patch.[9] After all, pellagra was not the first man-made hunger. The monoculture of cotton was not much different from the monoculture of sugar, which brought on a state of near starvation in Barbados in the seventeenth century, or the monoculture of rubber, which brought beriberi to the Amazon basin in the late nineteenth century. Captain Bligh had tried without success to solve the hunger problem of the sugar islands with breadfruit trees brought from the South Seas. Beriberi disappeared from the Amazon region only when the rubber bonanza economy vanished and the Amazon man was forced to go back to hunting, fishing, and harvesting wild fruits and nuts.[10] An agricultural and economic revolution was necessary to wipe out these nutritional diseases, and the same would be true of pellagra.

But Wheeler, like Goldberger, was no revolutionary. While his plans for influencing the minds of Southern bankers never came to much, he was more successful in his practical search for some simple food like cabbage or turnip greens to prevent pellagra. If tenant farmers were to be helped to help themselves, Wheeler observed, "any new and sudden departure must conform to the demands of a 'lazy man's' crop as much as possible."[11]

In Milledgeville, the search began again for a pellagra-preventing food. Wheeler decided to test canned vegetables, since fresh vegetables were not available year round and since vitamin

P-P or vitamin G was heat resistant and could not be destroyed by canning. He assumed that the fresh product would be as good or better. Tests ran for a year and, like the first ones, could be described only as dietary monotony. Those groups testing spinach ate it twice a day, every day, all year. The same was true of turnip greens, beans, and onions. Results of the tests fulfilled Wheeler's best hopes. Turnip greens, which grew almost as easily as weeds in the garden patch, were found to be a good source of the pellagra-preventive factor. They were cheap and they were available in the early spring, the season when they were most needed. Wheeler thought a little well-directed effort on the part of local health officials could boost the consumption of this Southern favorite, a hope which was eventually fulfilled. Spinach was less effective, although it contained some of the pellagra-preventive factor. Mature onions and green beans did not work at all; neither did lettuce or green onions. Mustard greens and green cabbage afforded some protection, but not so much as collards, kale, lean pork shoulder, green peas, and peanut meal, all of which joined turnip greens as completely protective foods. Pork shoulder and peanut meal were especially rich sources, with the virtues of the latter enhanced by its economy.[12]

Wheeler's practical approach to the pellagra problem was timely. Statistics on pellagra in the 1920s belied the national era of prosperity. Certainly in 1928 and 1929, there was not a chicken in every pot in the South. Rather, it seemed the Southern poor did not even get the neck. In 1928, pellagra caused almost as many deaths as typhoid fever; the Surgeon General called it the "most menacing single nutritional disease." Climbing rapidly after 1925, pellagra deaths reached a peak in Arkansas, Louisiana, and Tennessee in 1927, in South Carolina and Mississippi in 1928, in Georgia, Florida, and Virginia in 1929, and in North Carolina, Oklahoma, and Texas in 1930. Mortality from pellagra in the South jumped 58 percent in the five years from 1924 through 1928. The death figures told but part of the story. The Public Health Service figured there were 100 cases for every 3 deaths reported. This put the case rate at 170,000 in 1927 and at more than 200,000 during the next three years.[13]

When pellagra is considered as an essentially rural disease, the reason for this rise becomes clear. This was a time of agricultural depression. From the beginning of the decade, farmers were pinched for money, and by 1929 conditions were distressing. Not only was money short; so was food. The number of beef cattle in the South, for example, dropped by 24 percent from 1920 to 1928. The number of cows and heifers kept for milk also declined during the decade by slightly more than 6 percent; and even the ranks of the hardy porker were depleted. Tennessee had fewer than half the number of swine at the end of the 1920s that it had at the beginning. The failure of the South to do well with livestock was blamed on inadequate pasturage.[14]

Why the South with its copious rainfall, good soil, and a climate permitting work all year should be agriculturally poor baffled many thinking Southerners. Among these was the outspoken South Carolina conservationist James H. Rice. He blamed the "sickening mess" of agriculture in South Carolina on politics. Clemson College, he claimed, had been turned from the agricultural school it once was into a political institution because politics could not be allowed to suffer "no matter what happens to side-issues like farming." In Rice's opinion there were only four things which the South Carolina intellect comprehended: politics, cotton, horses, and religion. "Beyond these it ceases to function." Certainly, the South Carolina intellect was not devoting itself to food production. Rice knew of but two smokehouses on the whole South Carolina coast. Like George Washington, Rice thought that no people was happy until their food was abundant and cheap.[15]

In 1930, South Carolinians were still planting cotton, although the acreage had declined 2.7 percent annually from 1920 to 1929. *The Spartanburg Journal* accepted South Carolina's interest in cotton as right and natural. "What is needed just now is not so much the doctrine of 'reduced cotton acreage;' that is futile; the farmer is going to have as much if not more land in cotton this year as ever heretofore. But he should be informed how to grow more cotton at reduced cost per pound." By late summer 1930, however, the American Cotton Association was advocating a reduction of 15 million acres. Wheeler hoped the slump in the price of cotton in the early 1930s would be severe enough to curb the Southerner's interest in cotton altogether. The more unprofitable cotton production became, the more inclined Southerners would be to plant food crops. He believed the pellagra problem would solve itself if the price of cotton should stabilize itself at below five cents or above fifteen cents a pound.[16]

While pellagra may have been more prevalent in the rural areas, it was more conspicuous in the mill villages. Prevalence of the disease there in 1930 and 1931 was used by the American Federation of Labor's Southern Organizing Campaign as a wedge to organize labor in the Southern mills. *The American Federationist* made a survey of Southern mill villages and reported the average man working in the mills full time earned only $12.77 a week, of which $11.44 should go for food if a family of five was to be fed adequately. With rent to pay and clothing to buy, obviously it was impossible to spend so much at the grocery. Pellagra followed. Education on diet would help, *The Federationist* observed, but "even education cannot make bread out of a stone."[17]

In North Carolina in 1930, the year pellagra reached its postwar peak in that state, workers went on strike after wages were cut for the third time in eight months. *The American Labor Banner* reported that a pay increase of 20 percent plus steady work for North Carolina's half-million industrial population was necessary if pellagra were to be wiped out. There were 20,000 cases of it among the state's industrial population. Mill women asked how they could buy meat and milk and vegetables for their families on incomes of $6 or $7 a week. The money in their pay envelopes was not enough to buy food that would keep them in even moderate health.[18]

Labor was bitter about low pay, long hours, and the total lack of workmen's compensation. Southern workers put in about one-and-a-half times as many hours for half the weekly wage of New England operatives. Loom fixers in New England, for example, earned from $40 to $45 for a forty-hour week, while the same job in a South Carolina mill brought only $18 to $20 for sixty to sixty-five hours of work. The campaign to organize labor was fairly successful. Some unions were formed in the Carolinas and in Virginia, but, more important, the public became more sympathetic to the plight of the mill worker. Some educators began to laud the purposes of the AFL, and some ministers preached labor sermons and invited workers to hold meetings in their churches. The public showed a friendlier attitude, with popular opinion in North Carolina strongly supporting the strikers' demands for restoration of their old wages. The Cotton Textile Institute, an organization of manufacturers, responded to the pressure from AFL and mounting public opinion by eliminating night work for women in the mills. They said it was to stabilize production. Labor was jubilant and credited its success to focusing public attention on the social and economic evils of the textile industry. Only then did the industry realize that management of cotton textiles was a matter of public interest.[19]

Not only the textile strikes but a natural disaster brought pellagra to the nation's attention in 1930–1931. This was the drought that stretched across the nation from Pennsylvania and Ohio to Texas and Oklahoma. Extensive relief operations were needed in twenty-three states, many of them in the South. The Red Cross distributed food, served hot lunches in schools, and gave away yeast by the ton to those who had pellagra. This was but a reinforcement of the yeast-distribution program begun in the Mississippi flood area of 1927, a program which was continued there after the waters subsided and which quickly spread to neighboring states. By 1930, yeast was distributed regularly throughout the South. Equally important were the thousands of packages of garden seeds distributed to people in the drought area. New gardens put the pellagra-control program on the firmest foundation it had ever known.[20]

Garden seeds given away by the Red Cross sparked a grow-your-own-food campaign. The Red Cross first encouraged gardening in 1927 and 1928 when it gave away 120,000 packages of seed to people in the flood region. Seeds were distributed not so much to control pellagra as simply to alleviate the food shortage, but the resulting gardens served both purposes. The drought of 1930–1931 afforded a much larger test for the value of home gardens. The first seeds were used for fall gardens, which were started in 1930 as soon as rain came. Seeds were distributed in August to farmers in Arkansas, Kentucky, Louisiana, Mississippi, Oklahoma, and Texas. The packages contained seeds for crops farmers had never planted before and opened their eyes to new possibilities. Rye, for instance, replaced wheat and oats for late pasturage and made it possible to extend cultivation to freezing weather. In Mississippi, the help was desperately needed. People there had to contend that year not only with a drought, a poor cotton crop, and ruinously low prices, but with a bank collapse as well. One-third of the banks in the state were closed.[21]

The next spring the Red Cross gave away 611,000 assorted packages of garden seed. Each package contained from thirteen to eighteen varieties of vegetables suitable for a particular region and so selected that they provided food throughout the season. There were four pounds of seed in each package, enough for a garden a quarter-acre to a half-acre in size. For Southern gardens, the packages contained sixteen varieties: beans, beets, cabbage, carrots, corn, lettuce, kale, mustard, tomatoes, turnips, squash, onions, peas, spinach, okra, and collards. At least half of these were pellagra-preventive foods. Each package came complete with a pamphlet, *Home Gardening in the South,* which gave simple gardening instructions. Soon there were more gardens growing in the drought area than there had ever been before. People who had depended on cotton or another cash crop for trading at the grocery store discovered they could raise part of their own food. Some of the farmers embraced gardening enthusiastically, and men who had never grown food for themselves soon had giant-sized turnips or armloads of carrots and beets to show off to their neighbors. The new enthusiasm for gardening was accompanied by a new enthusiasm for home canning. Home Demonstration agents worked harder than ever to teach people how to can garden vegetables for winter use. Some statistics from Texas give an indication of their success. In 1930, there were 11 million glass and tin containers sold for home canning in Texas. In 1931, there were 30 million, and, in 1932, 50 million.[22]

As the depression deepened, the Red Cross had to curtail its yeast and garden seed programs, and the rate of decrease in pellagra, a decline which had been underway since 1931, slowed. In one state in which the Red Cross discontinued both programs in 1932 thinking that local initiative would take over, pellagra began to increase again, so the distribution of yeast was resumed. Unfortunately, the half million pounds of yeast which the Red Cross distributed in the decade after the Mississippi flood was not enough to meet the need. From 1933 to 1936, yeast was given only to those who needed it most; some pellagrins begged for a package of it when they became ill.[23]

On occasion local initiative did take over. Such was the case in Bell County, Kentucky, which Wheeler visited in the spring of 1932. This observation trip renewed his conviction that the key to pellagra control was education and publicity. In Bell County, where an intensive antipellagra campaign had been conducted by the local health department for many months, Wheeler could find only a few pellagrins. In Kentucky's Whitley County, where the people knew little or nothing about pellagra, there were several hundred victims. The economic conditions of the two counties were similar, and in both the people lived mainly on the basic diet of meat, meal, and molasses. In Bell County, however, health department officials had been busy, and the press was active in the antipellagra campaign. A pellagra clinic was conducted twice a week there by health officials. The homemakers club featured discussions on diet. Home production of vegetables was encouraged; yeast was distributed. The local paper printed diet instructions in language simple enough for anybody to understand: "Some families only eat fat meat, corn bread and molasses. The children in such families stay home from school, Sunday school, and church. The grown-ups feel too tired to work. In the spring the people usually come down with pellagra. Where families eat milk, potatoes, cabbage, greens, other vegetables and fruits every day . . . the children will not miss school . . . and the grown-ups will not feel too sick to work."[24] If some complained that pellagra-preventing foods were too expensive, the *Pineville Sun* pointed out that salmon cost only ten cents a can and four cans of tomatoes could be had for twenty-five cents.

The absence of pellagra in Bell County proved that the disease need not haunt a community, not even a seriously depressed one. The bituminous coal fields in Bell and Harlan counties were depressed enough in 1932 for the Friends Service Committee to move into the area to serve lunch to some 3,000 school children. Committees of reformers from New York, headed by Theodore Dreiser and Waldo Frank, came to check on conditions in the county. And the area was the first in the country to be fully organized for relief work under President Hoover. All charitable organizations were merged in each community in the two counties under a general welfare committee. Yet Wheeler could not find any pellagra.[25]

That same spring Wheeler went to two coal mining communities in Pennsylvania, in Lackawanna and Luzerne counties. He could find but one case of pellagra there, and that was a baker with peculiar dietary habits. But the diet of miners in Pennsylvania was vastly different from that of miners of Kentucky. In Pennsylvania fresh milk was plentiful and cheap, and mining families used it freely. They also ate fresh meat and vegetables. While many miners in Kentucky were a "floating" population, those in Pennsylvania were more stable, owned their own homes, and kept gardens. "If the prevailing dietary of the pellagrous sections of the South could be built up to where it even approximates in diversity and adequacy, that prevailing in the poorest sections of the mining districts of Pennsylvania," Wheeler wrote the Surgeon General, "endemic pellgra would cease to be a problem in this country."[26]

Wheeler's plan for initiating a pellagra-control program in the South was through practical demonstration. He wanted to prove in just one rural area where pellagra was prevalent that the people themselves could develop a workable scheme which would get them well and keep them pellagra-free.[27] The program he proposed was never conducted. Instead of a practical demonstration in one area, the pellagra-control program took the form of a massive educational campaign in which logic, reasoning, and occasional cajolery were brought to bear on the peculiar problems of the Southern diet.

Throughout the South, health officials in the 1930s began preaching the new gospel of vitamins and good-biological-quality proteins, but they found that many Southerners were loath to give up the traditional diet of meat, meal, and molasses. Those who tried to change food habits by telling people to give up their old favorites were doomed to disappointment. Most successful programs concentrated instead on teaching people to add supplementary foods to these staples. Wheeler appreciated the plight of the poor farmer who was told to cut out the three-M's without being given a substitute he could afford, and new proponents of a good diet had to accept that position, too.

The campaign to get Southern tenants and sharecroppers to plant gardens proved that people would use fresh vegetables if they were available. Much of the educational effort, therefore, went toward the promotion of gardening. County and home demonstration agents emphasized it, and relief commissions set up during the depression years gave out garden seeds along with yeast. Increasingly doctors, nurses, schools, and newspaper editors took part in the educational campaign. Their efforts were especially effective in the mill villages of South Carolina where Goldberger had made his house-to-house surveys during World War I. There were nutrition workers in these villages by 1930 and everybody from the best educated to the most unlettered referred to a "balanced diet" as the cure for pellagra. Children sang health songs at school, and health officers visited the schools to lecture on nutrition. The statewide effort to combat pellagra in South Carolina was interesting in view of the long quarrel health officer Hayne had with Goldberger. In 1931, Hayne, working with an officer from the Public Health Service, conducted a campaign in twenty-four South Carolina counties, holding clinics and distributing more than twenty-three tons of yeast.[28]

Some serious dietary studies were conducted in the South in the late 1920s to determine specifically what the nutritional deficiencies were. It was found that the rural people in Georgia, for example, fell far short of getting the iron and calcium they needed. The calcium deficiency was attributed to the fact that rural Georgians derived less than 10 percent of their calories from milk and cream, or more than 23 percent below the best standards of nutrition. They had more than enough protein, but too much of it came from vegetable sources. The diet, as expected, had an abnormally high content of fats and sweets. The survey noted that the average production of foods on the farm was not of sufficient variety to provide an adequate diet.[29]

A more detailed study of the Southern diet and its specific relation to pellagra was conducted by USDA officials in Lee County, South Carolina, in 1929. They came there when a young home demonstration agent, sent to the county in 1928, was shocked at the number of pellagrins she saw. On her second day on the job she found sixteen. She described the situation to the state office at Winthrop College, where an official from the Bureau of Home Economics in Washington happened to be visiting the day her letter arrived. Federal officials were looking for a likely spot for a study. Commercial firms were asked to donate food. One observer described the pellagrins of Lee County as isolated in poverty-ridden homes with bare, rough floors, the space dominated by two or three beds in each room. Mantels were filled with a variety of patent medicines "whose appeal has been made effective for the credulous, careless, and vascillating"; old bureaus were covered with snuff boxes. "Perhaps it is foolish to expect either the physical or mental energy to make a home attractive from these people who from the time they could walk and wear a sack over the shoulder were in the fields picking cotton from day-light until darkness. On Sundays they needed rest and recreation. For recreation they indulged in crude diversions, less immoral than unmoral."[30]

In the Lee County test were two groups of farm families: those who were so poor that they were likely to get pellagra unless they were given some supplementary foods, and those who were well-off enough to provide an adequate diet for themselves. Pellagra-preventing foods were distributed to the first group and sharply reduced the incidence of the disease. More interesting were the results of the study among those families who did not require aid. Some of these had woefully inadequate diets in spite of the fact that they could afford a better one. Their calorie-rich diets (as many as 4,794 a day) were heavy with starches, fats, and sugar; they contained but little protein. Those families who kept themselves pellagra-free had more than two cups of milk, three ounces of fruits or vegetables, and three ounces of lean meat for each person a day. The only way most of these rural families could provide themselves with such luxury when milk was ten cents a quart and steak thirty-five cents a pound was to produce food at home.[31]

There were many obstacles that stood in the way of securing an adequate diet for the masses of the South. A shortage of

refrigeration to keep meat fresh in the summertime was one
of these, but more important was the widespread opposition
on the part of many farmers to gardening or keeping a cow,
an opposition bred by a lifetime of cultivating cotton and corn.
There would have been little need for health officials to dabble
so much in agriculture if the economy had been differently organized and if there had been enough community dairies and
truck farms to supply the need. But this was not the case, and,
until there was basic economic change, the Red Cross and health
agencies engaged in stop-gap measures like lending a cow to
pellagra victims in times of distress.[32]

One of the ways by which health officials, both state and
federal, hoped to change dietary habits in the South was through
the publication of pamphlet guides to better eating. There were
dozens of these, most of which concentrated on ways in which
the diet could be improved without extra cost. Many low-cost
diets were recommended, but there was an "emergency food
guide" for the three-M area. It was difficult to prepare a pamphlet that communicated the exact message health authorities
wished to convey. The Public Health Service objected to one
prepared by the USDA because it advocated a fixed diet that
could be dangerous in a simple and restricted ration. Any seemingly insignificant departure could lead to a serious deficiency.
There was a worse error in a Georgia bulletin which reported
that "meats, milk, eggs, green vegetables, fruits—these foods
are rich in vitamins, maybe too rich." The PHS was unaware
that any food was too rich in the pellagra-preventing vitamin.
There was also the problem of illiteracy. One example will
suffice. Almost 17 percent of the population of South Carolina
over the age of fifteen was illiterate in 1930. This was more
than triple the national average.[33]

There was much incentive to spread the word about good
nutrition. In 1927 it was estimated that one-fourth of the children in the United States were inadequately nourished. In rural
Kentucky, for example, fully 40 percent of the children had

poor nutrition and another 35 percent no better than fair. Malnutrition had its mental as well as its physical effects, and studies were published showing that poor food was directly responsible for much of the low intelligence among the laboring classes. In the South, where pellagra was the most obvious result of poor nutrition, knowledgeable observers began to blame the shiftlessness and laziness of the Southern sharecropper on multiple vitamin deficiencies and inadequate intake of iron and protein. Rarely were pellagra producing diets inadequate in P-P vitamin only. Even Henry Ford climbed on the nutrition bandwagon, asserting that most crimes and wrongful actions were "the result of wrong mixtures in the stomach" and urging ministers to preach the gospel of nutrition from their pulpits.[34]

The educational campaign, along with a combination of other forces, sent the South's pellagra rate downward in the 1930s. From the peak year of 1928, the number of deaths from pellagra declined almost 50 percent by 1932. It continued to drop almost steadily after that, though not so rapidly. By 1935, the number of deaths from pellagra was very nearly the same as it had been ten years earlier when the disease began its precipitate rise. By 1940, with a dramatic new treatment available, the number of deaths was 77 percent lower than it had been in 1928.[35]

A drop in the incidence of pellagra in time of depression would seem to contradict Goldberger's theory that pellagra went up when prosperity went down. Actually, his theory still stood. Goldberger did not blame pellagra on poverty per se, but rather on poverty in combination with the unavailability of nutritious food. For various reasons there was more food available in the South in these very lean years than there had been when cotton was in its heyday. In those places where market outlets were closed to a staple commodity, farmers turned to producing food for home use. A survey in the postdepression years showed farmers were growing more garden truck. This was especially true in the South where owners, belatedly, decided it was cheaper for tenants to grow food than to furnish it. The Red

Cross gardens helped and so did the distribution of yeast, which, once begun by the states, was continued for more than twenty years.[36]

The coming of the New Deal with the inauguration of President Franklin D. Roosevelt in March 1933 was also a factor in the declining incidence of pellagra. The food relief program, administered first by the Federal Emergency Relief Administration, brought food to the South's hungry. Some of the surplus commodities were as familiar as cornmeal, but some, like graham flour and grapefruit juice, were strange to Southern tastes. The food relief program did not instigate a rapid decline in pellagra. Incidence of the disease dropped only slightly from 1933 to 1936 when more food was distributed for relief than ever before, but the new interest the government showed in the welfare of the common man was not without its effect. Indirectly, the creation of new jobs in agencies like the Civilian Conservation Corps helped, as did the new interest in restoring the land to a semblance of its old fertility. Creation of the Tennessee Valley Authority and the Rural Electrification Association hastened the spread of refrigeration across the South. Cold storage lockers appeared in many places where they had been unknown, helping to make food available at a low cost.[37]

The new start in life for tenants envisioned in the creation of the Resettlement Administration in 1935 did not bring the desired results, but its successor, the Farm Security Administration, created in 1937, made some real progress in teaching people how to live a little better. Under the direction of a Southerner, Dr. Will Alexander, the FSA launched a practical program, which concentrated on providing needy tenants with such prosaic items as a wagon, a mule, and cookstove. Provision of a wagon and a mule was based on the premise that a man could not get along in a modern age without some wheels under him; the cookstove made it possible for women who had never cooked on anything but the hearth to expand their culinary horizons. The FSA put up woven wire fences around garden patches to keep out the mule, and it taught people how to grow vegetables much as the Red Cross had done during the drought. It also provided pressure cookers so that surplus from the new gardens could be canned for winter use. These were soon dubbed "precious cookers" by many women who took to canning with a will and put up everything in sight, even catfish. The Resettlement Administration and the Farm Security Administration were programs in mass adult education. As Alexander said, "It was supervised credit plus adult education. There were hundreds of thousands of these people, and the interesting thing is that eighty-five percent of the total expenditure of FSA came back, once they got on their feet."[38] These workers had a broader interest than pellagra control, of course, but since pellagra was but a symbol of deeper social and economic problems, the mark of the butterfly began to disappear when basic conditions of life in the South changed.

This was the practical approach. It was in the tradition of Goldberger who for years urged tenants to keep a cow, and of Wheeler who found in ordinary turnip greens and collards a rich source of the essential pellagra-preventing vitamin. Wheeler had not given up the idea of proving in a demonstration that pellagra could be wiped out of a county by the bootstrap method of helping people to help themselves. In the spring of 1937, with the cooperation of the Red Cross, he thought he had his chance. Plans were made to set up demonstrations in one county in Tennessee, Arkansas, and Mississippi. Searches of each county were to be made for pellagra cases who would be put under a doctor's care; yeast would be distributed; gardens would be planted. On May 7, Wheeler and his associates from the PHS and the Red Cross set out from Memphis for Sunflower County, Mississippi, heart of the delta plantation region where pellagra had long been as familiar as cotton growing in the fields. They drove all day but found so few cases that the plan for a practical demonstration had to be abandoned.[39] In that one county at least, it was no longer necessary.

9

Victory

SPRING GARDENS, new cookstoves, and rows of canned vegetables on pantry shelves were a beginning, but final victory over pellagra came from advances in science and a basic change in the Southern economy. The 1930s brought the first; the 1940s and World War II brought the second.

There was fresh thinking about pellagra in these years, and new ideas about it came tumbling from hospitals and university laboratories. While the Public Health Service devoted itself primarily to a practical application of Goldberger's work, the search went on elsewhere for the specific element that was missing in the pellagrin's diet. It was at the University of Wisconsin where so much of the early important work on nutrition had been done that the nutritive "X" of pellagra was found. Scientists in the department of agricultural chemistry there hoped to isolate the antipellagra factor from liver extract, which many doctors lately had found valuable in treating pellagrins. They found what they were looking for almost by accident.

After months of working with puppies in which they had induced black tongue, they gave one of them some nicotinic acid which they had observed stimulated rat growth. A single dose of a commercial preparation gave a phenomenal response. The appetite improved immediately; the animal began growing again. Similar results were obtained with three other dogs. Wisconsin scientists then isolated nicotinic acid amide from liver extract and found that it, too, very effectively cured black tongue. Dr. Conrad A. Elvehjem and his associates reported their results in a simple letter to the editor of the *Journal of the American Chemical Society,* the writers observing in a bit of understatement that the possibility of a deficiency of nicotinic acid as the cause of black tongue was "most interesting."[1]

Elvehjem had grown up with nutrition work at Wisconsin. As a child in grade school he knew about the work of Stephen M. Babcock. As a student at that university in the 1920s, he had worked with E. B. Hart, one of those who had worked on the famous single-ration experiment with cows. He wrote his senior thesis under Dr. Harry Steenbock, best known for his discovery of adding vitamin D to foods through irradiation. As a graduate student at the University of Cambridge, he worked with enzymes. From England, he brought back to his Wisconsin laboratory a Warburg apparatus, one of the first available, and with this he explored how vitamins functioned. The mystery that had long surrounded vitamins began to disappear when specific ones were isolated and their chemical nature established.[2]

With Elvehjem's discovery, nicotinic acid was added to the list of known vitamins as part of the B-complex. It had been but four years since vitamin B_1, the long-sought antineuritic factor was identified. In 1933, Dr. R. R. Williams of the Bell Telephone Laboratories finally isolated thiamine. It was a job he had started more than twenty years before as a young assistant to Captain Vedder in the Philippines when he had been handed a jar of brown liquid from rice polishings and told to study it. By 1936, just three years after he discovered thiamine, Williams had learned its structure and was able to synthesize it.

The letter announcing nicotinic acid as the antipellagra factor appeared in September 1937. There was an immediate reaction in the medical profession as physicians in many American cities initiated tests to determine safe dosages of nicotinic acid, and this done, began to treat their patients. Results everywhere were spectacular. Patients showed dramatic improvement, sometimes within hours. Nicotinic acid was hailed as a miracle healer. It was not only effective, but it was also cheap and easily administered.

There was widespread optimism, this time well founded, that in nicotinic acid a cure for pellagra had been found. The *Southern Medical Journal,* which over a period of thirty years had included many pages of acrimonious debate over the pellagra question, commented editorially that a "hopeful but conservative" outlook could be taken on the prevention of pellagra by means of this new vitamin. A group of thirty-nine well-known American scientists was so sure that nicotinic acid was the answer that it contributed to a fund to send it to Spain where pellagra had broken out as a result of the civil war. There was enough to treat 40,000 people, the first really large-scale test of the new remedy.[3]

Nicotinic acid was the key to the problem of pellagra, but effective as it was, it could not answer all the nutritional deficiency problems of the South. Pellagra was too frequently compounded with beriberi and other avitaminoses for the patient to rely on nicotinic acid alone. The condition doctors generally found in the field was one of multiple deficiencies all of which had to be treated. Too little nicotinic acid was the most critical shortage in the pellagrin's diet, but often, it was not the only factor missing. The introduction of nicotinic acid, however, sent the death rate from pellagra tumbling. In 1940, three years after it was introduced, there were 2,040 deaths from pellagra in the United States; by 1945, the figure dropped to 865. The case rate was cut, too, from almost 9,000 cases in 1940 to less than half that five years later. *The Commonweal* called the pellagra cure science at its best: "This will . . . work a beneficent revolution in the South, where the gain, personal and economic, from the restoration to health and working ability of a large section of the population, is indeed beyond computation."[4]

The beneficent revolution did not come overnight, and it was not nicotinic acid alone that finally brought it about. Good nutrition was a problem for the commonwealth. The need for government action in nutrition work had been pointed out in at least two famous reports in the 1930s. A study on the relation of diet to income in Britain showed that the new knowledge of nutrition coming at the same time as greatly increased powers of producing food created an entirely new situation demanding "economic statesmanship."[5] About the same time, a committee on nutrition of the League of Nations meeting in Geneva called for the establishment of national nutrition committees composed of people experienced in health, agriculture, economics, finance, and social welfare. Application of the newer knowledge of nutrition had only just begun. The league report said ultimate responsibility for its application rested with governments.[6]

Experts gathered at Geneva worked out a table, "The Geneva Standards," which set down nutrition requirements. They paid attention to vulnerable groups in the population most subject to malnutrition—children, pregnant women, nursing mothers, and the aged—and they dealt not only with calorie and protein needs but with nutrients the body could not synthesize. It was a bold venture, for only a few vitamins had been discovered and little, if anything, was known on how much of them a person required. But work done at Geneva did make it possible to estimate what a proper diet for an individual, a family, a city, an army, or a nation should be.[7]

The Geneva Standards were put to the test in World War II. What Andrew Mayer, French member of the league's committee on health, called the "marriage of food and agriculture" became a reality. Food rationing in many countries of the world was done on the basis of work done at Geneva. In Great Britain the results were striking. Despite the upheaval of the war, the diet of the British people actually improved, and infant mortality fell to lower levels than ever before. In the United States, agriculture adjusted dramatically to "nutritional planning." Within two years the United States had increased agricultural output by one-third and was feeding an additional 40 million people.[8]

A combination of forces revolutionized the Southern diet in the years after 1940. Food rationing in World War II inspired some people to buy and eat high protein foods, which they had never particularly wanted before, and increased employment and mobilization of the armed forces provided incomes large enough to purchase a better diet. Equally important, vitamins came into their own. "Vitamins Will Win the War" was suggested as the World War II successor to the "Food Will Win the War" slogan of World War I.[9] It did not catch on, but the new emphasis on vitamins helped to spell the end of pellagra. Thanks to the wartime emergency, the vital B vitamins—including among others the antineuritic factor, thiamine, and the pellagra-preventive factor, nicotinic acid—were increased in the diet in the form of enriched bread and flour. The staff of life, which had become a somewhat frail reed, was greatly strengthened. It became difficult to avoid vitamin B. It was said that if a man ate enough to stay alive, he was almost sure to get his quota.

Enrichment of bread and flour was the modern solution to a problem about which there had been an occasional protest in America for more than a hundred years. Sylvester Graham, nineteenth-century dietary reformer, was such a vocal advocate of whole-wheat bread that his name became synonymous with the product. Scientific advances in the 1930s made it possible to make white bread as wholesome as Graham's whole wheat. Synthetic thiamine and commercially available nicotinic acid could be added to flour at the mill or to bread at the bakery.

Addition of the B vitamins to white bread was not the first effort to enrich it. In the 1920s, many bakers began to improve the nutritional quality of white bread by adding skim milk solids to it. At the suggestion of nutrition expert Elmer V. McCollum, most commercial bakers began adding 6 percent nonfat milk solids to their product.[10] The first vitamin to be added to bread, flour, milk, and other products was vitamin D. In 1924, Dr. Harry Steenbock at the University of Wisconsin discovered a way to build bone-building vitamin D artificially. In Paul De Kruif's phrase, he "trapped the sun's rays" by exposing food to ultraviolet radiation. By 1925 he demonstrated his discovery with milk, meat, cereals, flour, oils, and corn. In response to this discovery, the Wisconsin Alumni Research Foundation was established that year to promote research by commercial development of scientific discovery. Two years later the WARF awarded the first contract for irradiation of foods to Quaker Oats Company, which obtained exclusive rights to the process in the manufacture of cereal foods. In 1929 and 1930 several foreign firms, an American yeast manufacturer, and one of the nation's largest bread companies signed agreements with the foundation. In the next decade, enough research was conducted to show that irradiation had beneficial effects, and Steenbock's process was adapted to the commercial milk field. By 1936 irradiated milk was available almost everywhere in the United States. The foundation moved slowly, conducting extensive clinical tests, in order not to antagonize the medical profession whose friendship it deemed crucial to the successful commercial application of the Steenbock patent.[11]

The American Medical Association was receptive to the fortification program. Its Council on Foods and Nutrition and its Council on Pharmacy and Chemistry in 1938 agreed that it was desirable to add vitamins to certain staple foods. They suggested that 400 units of vitamin D be added per quart of milk and that enough vitamin A be added to butter substitutes to equal the vitamin A in butter. The Food and Nutrition Board of the National Research Council reported in 1939 that it would regard with favor the addition of thiamine and other nutrients to white bread and flour, and the AMA agreed. That same year, Dr. Williams, the synthesizer of thiamine, told cereal chemists meeting in New York City it would be "suicidal" for food industries "to blink at scientific facts which will presently become common knowledge." The industry had to make staple products more nearly equivalent in nutritive value to the whole seed as it was consumed by primitive man. They could do it either by adding synthetic materials or by retaining the original nutritive components.[12]

The campaign to add vitamins to bread and flour picked up speed in 1940. That summer as the Battle of Britain raged, the British government proposed to fortify flour with synthetic thiamine as part of the war effort. At the same time, in the United States the Committee on Medicine of the National Research Council advised the reinforcement with thiamine of all white flour purchased for the military forces, and the Food and Drug Administration scheduled public hearings on nutritional standards that should be set for white flour. By early January 1941, the Millers' National Federation was ready to adhere to these standards. Although nutritive elements had been added to bread for almost two decades, primarily through the use of irradiated yeast, the addition of synthetic nutrients to flour was described as the first major change in milling since the introduction of the roller mill, and it was ranked as one of the few major developments in an ancient industry. At first the millers wanted to add only thiamine, but agreed to add niacin (the abbreviated name given nicotinic acid), too. The addition of riboflavin, still another B vitamin, was to come later.[13] "It looks now as if the war will do more for the general consumption of needed vitamins than all the preaching of the nutrition experts," *The New York Times* commented editorially. Vitamins were so cheap that they added but little to the cost, about three cents for a twelve-pound sack of flour and two-tenths of one cent for a one-pound loaf of white bread.[14]

President Roosevelt launched a massive attack on malnutrition by calling a National Nutrition Conference for Defense in late

May 1941 to work out a plan for strengthening the nation by strengthening her people. Good food was the key. Enrichment of bread was a step toward a better diet for every American, but in itself was not enough. At the conference Paul V. McNutt, administrator of the Federal Security Agency and coordinator of health, welfare, and related defense activities, warned that enrichment was no "magic wand" which made bread a substitute for other food.[15]

The nutritional shortcomings of the South received special attention at the conference and a pledge that the whole nation would help to solve the problem. Surgeon General Thomas Parran reminded the delegates that from the Mississippi valley, the richest in the world, "we have exported the soil in the form of cotton, and created an economy of poverty, of tenancy, of pellagra, of anemia, and of hookworm. The rest of the country must help to restore and the job will take long years." The conference approved a yardstick by which an adequate diet in the South or any other part of the nation could be measured. This yardstick was the list of minimum daily requirements of various dietary essentials drawn up by the National Research Council. For the first time there was a fairly accurate way to determine who was and who was not underfed. Acute symptoms of diseases like pellagra and beriberi were not an accurate enough gauge. Only one undernourished person in ten wore such a visible badge of a poor diet. The conference recommended to the President that America build a stronger people through the "conquest of hunger—not only the obvious hunger that man has always known, but the hidden hunger revealed by the modern knowledge of nutrition."[16]

The yardstick adopted at the conference had been worked out by a special committee of the National Research Council's Food and Nutrition Board. It took about a year for standards to be set. One of the committee's more difficult problems was to determine the amount of niacin needed. Since there were no human studies to go on, the Committee applied Elvehjem's rule for rats: ten times as much niacin as thiamine is required. They also specified the addition of another B vitamin, riboflavin, and iron, as well as calcium and vitamin D on an optional basis.[17]

The nation's millers quickly embraced the idea of enriching flour. The long and fruitful experience of bakers with irradiated yeast made it comparatively easy. There was no compulsion about it at first, but the number of millers and bakers who complied with the recommendations was so great that, by January 1943, 75 percent of all white bread was being enriched. That was the month the newly created War Food Administration issued its first order, one requiring that vitamins and minerals be added to all bakers' white bread. The order was issued under emergency war powers, which ended with the Japanese surrender in 1945, but by that time numerous states had initiated legislation requiring the enrichment of all white flour, bread, and cornmeal. South Carolina led the way. It was the first state to require by law the enrichment of white bread and flour.[18]

Because of technical difficulties there was no mandatory enrichment of flour during the war. Could the federal government order flour enriched when used for state-operated institutions? Should all baker's flour, even that used for crackers and cakes, be enriched? The effect of omitting mandatory enrichment of flour most affected the hot bread belt of the South, those who lived in institutions, and those who ate most of their meals out. Except in states like South Carolina with mandatory enrichment programs, relatively little of the cheapest grades of flour that went into the mouths of the most poorly fed was enriched.[19]

In spite of these obvious shortcomings, overall the enrichment program was a success. After it was started, the average American diet contained twice as much thiamine, riboflavin, and niacin as before. Enrichment played a part in the disappearance of the deficiency diseases pellagra and beriberi. Reports from New York City's Bellevue Hospital showed that these two diseases decreased "markedly and unmistakably" during 1942 and

1943, the period when enriched white bread and flour became universally available in the city. And nicotine, once a drag on the market, became rather scarce. It was the best source for nicotinic acid for which there was unprecedented demand. Some 300,000 pounds of it were used in 1942 to fortify flour.[20]

There were problems in the early enrichment program. So many people thought enrichment was required by the government that they assumed all bread and flour was enriched and did not ask for it specifically. Enriched flour and bread cost slightly more, and so did not sell as well. There were some people, too, who thought the milling and baking industries were trying to make a profit off enrichment and so resisted pressure to ask for enriched products. The ghost of Sylvester Graham also hampered the enrichment program, for many people were convinced that whole-wheat bread was better than white bread, and some thought erroneously that any dark bread was whole wheat. A vast educational campaign had to be conducted to educate the public.[21] The task was undoubtedly easier than it might have been because the way had been paved by more than twenty years of talk about vitamins and because much of the public had become accustomed to the idea of irradiated foods in the 1930s. Still the task was difficult. Millions of leaflets and posters were distributed explaining what enrichment meant and why it was important. People had to be taught, too, that they washed away vitamins when they rinsed off enriched rice or grits before cooking it (the B vitamins are water soluble).

Education of Southern tenants and sharecroppers was the most difficult of all. The new nutrition workers in the South ran into the same problems Goldberger faced in trying to change dietary patterns. For one thing, most of the posters, leaflets, and radio programs reached only white women of the owner or long-term sharecropper classes, not those who really needed help most. And for another, basic attitudes about food remained unchanged. The Southern belief that Negroes needed less food than whites persisted.[22]

But the rapid urbanization of the South after the war changed Southern tastes. An increasing variety of foods was available. Better transportation, advances in technology, new methods of preserving foods, and a shift in the agricultural emphasis from cotton to beef and dairy cattle, peanuts and vegetables, all played a part in rapidly changing the section's dietary habits. When the one-crop system of agriculture began to fade, the force that dictated the peculiar meat, meal, and molasses diet was removed.

Two more pieces of the chemical puzzle of pellagra fell into place in 1945. Both came from the agricultural chemistry laboratory of the University of Wisconsin. Scientists there fed dogs on unenriched corn grits and found that corn in the diet "significantly increases" the nicotinic acid requirement. The more corn the diet contained the more nicotinic acid was required. Other dogs, fed on a milk and mineral diet, which contained relatively much less nicotinic acid, grew better. While corn made more nicotinic acid necessary, milk definitely decreased the requirement. This was the first scientific proof that there was something valid in the old argument of the Zeists that pellagra was caused by eating corn. Indeed, they were right.[23]

A few months later, another bit of the riddle was solved. It proved that Goldberger and Tanner had hold of a significant bit of truth twenty-four years before when they said that pellagra might be caused by an amino acid deficiency. Their spectacular results in treating pellagrins with the amino acid tryptophan were not accidental. In the spring of 1945 Wisconsin scientists, pursuing their work on grits and pellagra, added tryptophan to a test diet laden with corn. There was a dramatic growth response. Although the relationship between tryptophan and nicotinic acid was obscure at first, time revealed that both man and animals under the right conditions can convert tryptophan into nicotinic acid. Pellagra could represent a deficiency of both.[24]

By this time, pellagra had been part of the Southern scene for almost four decades. It had probably been present, but unrecognized, for much longer, perhaps as much as a century or more. Rooted in the South's monotonous dietary pattern, pellagra increased as that diet became more restricted. The advent of highly milled corn and wheat, which composed more than half the total diet of many Southern poor, may have hastened the day when the disease burst into the open after a long incubation.

Pellagra appeared on the Southern scene amidst a blaze of publicity. Its rather rapid disappearance in the years after 1945 went almost unnoticed. The South that spawned it was no more. Cotton tenancy collapsed and the company-owned cotton-mill towns disappeared. People from the rural areas and those from mill villages, pellagra's chief victims, shopped in supermarkets just as their city neighbors did. The three-M's gave way to variety.

For those whose food habits did not change with the changing times, synthetic vitamins added to flour, cornmeal, and grits provided at least a partial shield against almost-sure illness. Some smaller grocery stores continued to cater to the three-M taste with window displays of a "$5.98 Payday Special": a sack of meal, one of flour, another of grits, a bucket of lard, a pound of coffee, and a couple of cans of corn and tomatoes. But this was an echo of the past, a fleeting reminder of a way of life that fostered poverty and disease.

10

Epilogue

THE FACE OF HUNGER has changed in the South. It no longer wears the mask of the butterfly. Its new look can hardly be distinguished from that of hunger in the North or West. Everywhere the hungry poor look the same, most often too thin, but occasionally too fat, because their diet is all starch and no protein. They are often sick; their eyes lack lustre; they have little energy. They are white and black. Many of them are women and children like those Joseph Goldberger saw as he tramped through the streets of South Carolina mill villages looking for telltale ugly red marks of pellagra. The South, which has lost its distinctiveness as a region in so many ways, has also lost its distinctive mark of hunger. The butterfly caste is gone.

But it is not entirely gone, to be sure. It crops up often enough to remind one it could come back again. Senator Ernest F. Hollings found some pellagrins on his tour of shacks in Beaufort County, South Carolina, in 1969 along with cases of scurvy and rickets. In 1971 the state health officer of Maryland found pellagra in the mental hospitals of that state and blamed it on a legislative economy move which directed that seventy-two cents per day be spent for food instead of the minimum of one dollar considered necessary for an adequate diet. But most pellagrins have disappeared.

The one thing that has not changed about hunger in America since Goldberger's day is its politics. Hunger is still a thorny political issue. Goldberger, certainly not a politician, not even a social reformer, but just a doctor who saw a problem and knew how to solve it in the scientific sense, stumbled innocently into the politics of hunger in 1921. He thought he had but to call the nation's attention to the problem and it would be solved. "We are feeding the Near East and the Far East but we are neglecting our own people right here at home," he said. President Harding, a political innocent insofar as hunger was concerned, responded immediately: "Famine and plague are words almost foreign to our American vocabulary, save as we have learned their meaning in connection with the afflictions of lands less favored and toward which our people have so many times displayed large and generous charity." In the furor that followed and amidst vehement denials that anybody was hungry in the South, the President backed away, and Goldberger went back to the laboratory.

In the last years of the 1960s when hunger in America again became an issue, there was almost a repeat performance of the 1921 episode insofar as charges and countercharges about hunger were concerned. Senator Hollings sought out the hungry poor in South Carolina and found them by the thousands. But South Carolinians were as defensive in the 1960s as they had been almost a half-century earlier. They denied that hunger existed; they accused the Senator of ruining the tourist industry; they called him a Communist. Congressman L. Mendel Rivers branded him "Hookworm Hollings." The Nebraska doctor, Donald Gatch, who moved to Beaufort and began to treat the hungry, and then testified about the seriousness of the problem both in county forums and at the state capital, became such a controversial figure he had to leave town.

In the spring of 1969, President Richard Nixon, responding to the agitation over hunger, made a statement that might have been copied from the Harding file: "So accustomed are most of us to a full and balanced diet that until recently, we have thought of hunger and malnutrition as problems only in less fortunate countries. . . . That [they] should persist in a land such as ours is embarrassing and intolerable."

The food stamp program which followed has helped some to alleviate the problem, but not very much. Neither food stamps nor distribution of surplus commodities has been much more effective in meeting the problem of hunger in America than Goldberger's campaign to change the pattern of Southern agriculture. Politically it is safer and more popular to help hungry foreigners than hungry Americans.

The fight against pellagra was in many ways a preview of the current struggle against hunger. Pellagrins were isolated in mill villages or in rural areas down winding dirt roads most people never saw. The modern poor are equally isolated in the same rural areas or in city slums, places hardly visible to most Americans because, as Vice-President Agnew remarked, "If you've seen one, you've seen them all." Politically, hunger is almost as invisible in America as it was a half-century ago, but not quite. The Senate's Select Committee on Nutrition and Human Needs helps to keep the issue of hunger before the American public. Such a committee would have been unthinkable in 1921.

Pellagra continued to be a spectre in the South years after the cure was known because most Southerners refused to believe it existed. Hunger persists because most Americans do not believe it is there. Just as the presence of pellagra cast doubt on the prosperity and virtue of the New South, the presence of hunger denies the validity of the American dream. It is too painful an idea to be borne. It is easier and more comfortable to deny all charges of hunger in America.

Goldberger would understand the dilemma of those who believe the nation's hunger problem could be solved if only the American people could see that the problem exists. He would understand, too, how difficult is the task of convincing well-fed Americans that people a few blocks or, at most, a few miles from them are hungry. "I doubt if they are any worse off in Belgium," he wrote of the hungry people of South Carolina mill villages at the height of World War I. "Some day this will be realized and something done to correct it."

In many ways America's poor are still waiting.

Notes

Chapter 1
A New Scourge for the South

1. H. F. Harris, "A Case of Ankylostomaisis Presenting the Symptoms of Pellagra," *Transactions, Medical Association of Georgia* (1902), 220–227.

2. George H. Searcy, "An Epidemic of Acute Pellagra," *Transactions of the Medical Association of the State of Alabama* (1907), 387–392.

3. Ibid.

4. James W. Babcock, "How Long Has Pellagra Existed in the United States?" in *Transactions of the National Association for the Study of Pellagra* (Columbia, S.C.: The R. L. Bryan Co., 1914), 14 (hereafter cited as *Tr., NASP*).

5. *65th Annual Report of the Georgia State Sanitarium* (1908), 21–22.

6. *66th Annual Report of the Georgia State Sanitarium* (1909), 28, 45, 56.

7. *Report of the Board of Administrators of Louisiana Hospital for Insane* (1910), 15–16.

8. George A. Zeller, "Pellagra: Its Recognition in Illinois," *Transactions of the National Conference on Pellagra* (Columbia, S.C.: The State Co., Printers, 1910), 47–52 (hereafter cited as *Tr., Natl. Conf.*).

9. M. B. Young, "Pellagra in Children," *Tr. Natl. Conf.*, 267–268; United States Public Health Service, General File, No. 1648, Boxes 150–151, National Archives, Washington, D.C. (hereafter cited as NA).

10. There are many vivid descriptions of the disease in medical journals. Nearly every doctor who wrote on pellagra described it in some detail. Among the more readily accessible of these is Edward Jenner Wood, "The Appearance of Pellagra in the United States," *Journal of the American Medical Association* 53 (July 24, 1909): 274–282 (hereafter cited as *JAMA*).

11. James W. Babcock, "The Prevalence and Psychology of Pellagra," *American Journal of Insanity* 67 (January 1911): 537–538; C. H. Lavinder, *Pellagra, A Précis* (Washington: Government Printing Office, 1908), 11–14; James Babcock, "Medico-Legal Relations of Pellagra," *Tr., NASP,* 396–401; *The* (Milledgeville, Ga.) *Union Recorder,* March 19, 1912; *Report of the State Board of Health of Mississippi, 1915–1917,* 113.

12. J. W. Mobley, "Pellagra, Its Relation to Insanity and Certain Nervous Diseases," *Tr., Natl. Conf.,* 137.

13. Babcock, "How Long Has Pellagra Existed?" 17–18; *New York Times,* September 8, 1916, p. 13.

14. G. A. Wheeler, "A Note on the History of Pellagra in the United States," *Public Health Reports* 46 (September 18, 1931): 2226–2228 (hereafter cited as *PHR*); Mobley, "Pellagra, Its Relation to Insanity," 144.

15. Quoted in Cecilia C. Mettler, *History of Medicine* (Philadelphia: The Blakiston Co., 1947), 411–412.

16. Ralph Major, "Don Gaspar Casál, Francois Thiéry and Pellagra," *Bulletin of the History of Medicine* 16 (November 1944): 356–357; Fielding H. Garrison, *An Introduction to the History of Medicine,* 4th ed. (Philadelphia: W. B. Saunders Co., 1929), 368. Casal's classic book was *Historia Natural y Medica de la Principado de Asturias* (Madrid: Manuel Martin, 1762). Thiéry's account appeared in *Journal de Médecine, Chirugie et Pharmacie* 2 (1755): 337–346.

17. Major, "Don Gaspar Casál," 359; Goethe quoted in *JAMA* 59 (September 21, 1912): 959–960.

18. William H. Deaderick and L. Thompson, *Endemic Diseases of the Southern States* (Philadelphia: W. B. Saunders Co., 1916), 297; "Corn and Pellagra," *Review of Reviews* 41 (March 1910): 352; Edward Podolsky, "Joseph Goldberger and the Mysterious Hunger," *New York Journal of Medicine* 56 (1961): 2489; Joseph Goldberger, "The Relation of Diet to Pellagra," *JAMA* 78 (June 3, 1922): 1676; C. H. Lavinder, "The Aetiology of Pellagra," *New York Medical Journal* 90

(July 10, 1909): 56. For a complete account of the Zeist theory of the Italians, see George M. Niles, *Pellagra, An American Problem,* 2d ed. (Philadelphia: W. B. Saunders Co., 1916), 34–50, and Stewart R. Roberts, *Pellagra: History, Distribution, Diagnosis, Prognosis, Treatment, Etiology* (St. Louis: C. V. Mosby Co., 1913), 232–247.

19. James J. Wolfe, "Pellagra: The Causative Agent and the Method of Infection," *South Atlantic Quarterly* 9 (1910): 52–53. Wolfe, a professor at Trinity College (later Duke University) in North Carolina, tested the temperature of a corn cake cooking on top of the stove, checking it every two minutes for an hour. The highest temperature reached was only 178 degrees.

20. Francis Butler Simkins, *Pitchfork Ben Tillman, South Carolinian* (Baton Rouge: Louisiana State University Press, 1944), 463; Alvey A. Arlee to Secretary of Treasury, July 22, 1909, NA.

21. South Carolina State Board of Health, *Conference on Pellagra Held Under Auspices of the State Board of Health at the State Hospital for the Insane, Oct. 29, 1908* (Columbia: The State Co. Printers, 1909), 3–4.

22. Burton J. Hendrick, "The Mastery of Pellagra," *The World's Work* 31 (April 1916): 633–634; George Searcy, "Pellagra in the Southern States," *New Orleans Medical and Surgical Journal* 61 (December 1908): 423; Wood, "Appearance of Pellagra," 281–282; *The State* (Columbia, S.C.), November 11, 1909.

23. Quoted in *The Literary Digest* 39 (November 13, 1909): 827, and *The Literary Digest* 41 (October 8, 1910): 583; *Report, Louisiana State Board of Health, 1908–09,* 205–207. The reporter from *McClure's* gathered much information at a meeting of a special pellagra conference in Abbeville, S.C., August 6, 1909. Approximately 125 physicians attended this meeting and reported mortality from pellagra at 50 percent, with estimates as high as 70 percent.

24. *The State,* November 2, 1909.

25. Harry Frank Farmer, "The Hookworm Eradication Program in the South, 1909–1925" (Ph.D. diss., University of Georgia, 1970), 2–4, 31, 47, 124, 143; *The State,* November 4, 1909.

26. Quoted in Farmer, "Hookworm Eradication," 148–149.

27. F. M. Sandwith, "Introductory Remarks," *Tr., Natl. Conf.,* 19; Sandwith to Babcock, August 26, 1909, James Woods Babcock Papers, South Caroliniana Library, Columbia, S.C. (hereafter Babcock Papers, SC).

28. Lavinder to Wyman, July 8, 1909, NA. Members of the commission were Dr. John F. Anderson, Dr. Reid Hunt, Dr. C. H. Lavinder,

Dr. John D. Long, Dr. M. J. Rosenau, Dr. William White, and Dr. Nicholas Achuccaro.

29. Lavinder to Wyman, July 6, 1909, NA.

30. J. D. Long to Kerr, April 3, 1910, NA.

31. Long to Kerr, April 11, 1910, Long to Surgeon General, April 9, 16, 1910, a NA.

32. *The State,* November 3, 4, 5, 1909; *The Richmond* (Va.) *Journal,* November 5, 1909.

33. "Conference on Pellagra," *JAMA* 53 (November 13, 1909): 1670.

34. William S. Hall, "Psychiatrist, Humanitarian, and Scholar: James Woods Babcock, M. D.," *The Journal of the South Carolina Medical Association* (October 1970): 366; Walter Cheyne to Babcock, July 30, 1909, Babcock Papers, SC; "Report and Proceedings of Special Legislative Committee to Investigate the State Hospital for the Insane and State Park," *Reports and Resolutions of South Carolina* (1914), IV, 936.

35. Lavinder, "The Aetiology of Pellagra," 55; Lavinder, *Pellagra, A Précis,* 20.

36. B. T. Galloway to Walter Wyman, February 17, 1909, NA.

37. E. J. Watson, "Economic Factors of the Pellagra Problem in South Carolina," *Tr., Natl. Conf.,* 27–28; *Chicago Post,* quoted in Notebook, James Woods Babcock Papers, Library of the Medical University of South Carolina, Charleston (hereafter cited as Babcock Papers, Ch).

38. Quoted in *The Literary Digest* 41 (October 8, 1910): 583. Beer manufacturers denied the charge that beer was pellagra producing. No germ could withstand the heat of beer manufacture. See *The Literary Digest* 42 (March 4, 1911): 401–402.

39. E. J. Watson, "Economic Factors of the Pellagra Problem in the South," *Tr., Natl. Conf.,* 30; J. Swinton Whaley, "Personal Experience with Damaged Corn," *Tr. Natl. Conf.,* 199–201.

40. Carl L. Alsberg, "Agricultural Aspects of the Pellagra Problem in the United States," *New York Medical Journal* 90 (July 10, 1909): 51–53.

41. C. W. G. Rohrer, "Pellagra, Its Etiology, Pathology, Diagnosis and Treatment," *Tr., Natl. Conf.,* 96; J. S. DeJarnet, "Pellagra, the Corn Curse," *Tr. Natl. Conf.,* 288–292.

42. Lavinder, "The Prophylaxsis of Pellagra," ms., NA. Other measures taken by the Italian government to prevent the disease were the provision of cheap cooperative kitchens, the improvement of agriculture, and the education of the people. To cure pellagra, the government provided for free distribution of salt (a government monopoly in Italy),

the distribution of food either in homes or in sanitary stations, and the treatment of severe cases in hospitals.

43. Otis F. Black and Carl Alsberg, *The Determination of the Deterioration of Maize, with Incidental Reference to Pellagra,* Bureau of Plant Industry Bulletin 199 (Washington: Government Printing Office, 1910), 7–8, 12; Alsberg, "Agricultural Aspects of Pellagra," 54.

44. *Savannah* (Ga.) *Morning News,* August 24, 1911; *The Causation of Pellagra,* Bulletin, Georgia State Board of Health, Series 2, I (1912).

45. South Carolina, *Acts of South Carolina 1910,* Act No. 304, 613–622.

46. Quoted in Francis Robbins Allen, "Public Health Work in the Southeast, 1872–1941: The Study of a Social Movement" (Ph.D. diss., University of North Carolina, 1946), 351.

47. DeJarnet, "Pellagra, the Corn Curse," 293; J. W. Kerr, "Notes on Hematology of Pellagra," *Tr., Natl. Conf.,* 20; Lavinder, *Pellagra, A Précis,* 8–9; *The Daily Record* (Columbia, S.C.), n.d., clipping in Babcock Papers, Ch.

48. J. H. Taylor, "Sambon the Man and His Later Investigations of Pellagra," *Tr., NASP,* 69–72.

49. Quoted in *The Literary Digest* 41 (October 1, 1910), 789–790.

50. Stewart R. Roberts, "The Analogies of Pellagra and the Mosquito," *Tr., NASP.,* 291–296; Chilton Thorington, "Some Suggestions As to the Etiology of Pellagra," *Virginia Medical Semi-Monthly* 16 (July 21, 1911): 185–189.

51. *JAMA* 59 (November 23, 1912), 1917–1918; John L. Jelks, "The Etiology of Pellagra," *Southern Medical Journal* 5 (March 1912): 72–75 (hereafter cited as *SMJ*).

52. M. L. Ravitch, "A Plea for Earlier Diagnosis of Pellagra," *JAMA* 59 (July 6, 1912): 33–35.

53. *The State,* October 4, 1912. For later endorsements of the sugar-cane theory, see J. F. Yarbrough, "Pellagra: Its Etiology, Symptomatology and Treatment," *The Medical Record* (November 24, 1917), reprint, and Roy Blosser, "Some Observations Further Incriminating Sugar Cane Products as the Main Cause of Pellagra in the South," *SMJ* 8 (1915): 33–36. An account of Dr. Deeks's work in the tropics is included in Charles Morrow Wilson, *Ambassadors in White* (New York: Henry Holt & Co., 1942), 156–183.

54. Lavinder to Wyman, August 26, 1911, N. Musher to Emmet A. Jones, December 21, 1915, NA.

55. George C. Mizell, "Etiologic Factor and Recurrent Attacks of Pellagra," *Tr., NASP,* 297–304.

56. B. F. Taylor to Lavinder, June 17, 1911, Lavinder to Wyman, August 25, 1911, NA.

57. Lavinder to Wyman, June 23, August 26, 1911, NA.

58. A. B. Clark, "Diseases of the Eye in Pellagra," *Tr., Natl. Conf.,* 275–278.

59. "A Successful Attempt in Producing Pellagra in a Monkey," *SMJ* 6 (July 1913): 483–484.

60. C. H. Lavinder, "The Prevalence and Geographic Distribution of Pellagra in the United States," *PHR* 27 (December 13, 1912): 2077, 2087–2088. These eight states were Virginia, North Carolina, South Carolina, Georgia, Kentucky, Alabama, Mississippi, and Louisiana. These figures do not include pellagrins in insane asylums.

61. *67th Annual Report of the Georgia State Sanitarium* (1910), 20; Tennessee, State Board of Health, *Pellagra, A Report* (Nashville, 1911); "Pellagra," *JAMA* 57 (September 2, 1911): 827; *Greensboro* (N.C.) *News,* January 5 (?), 1914, clipping in NA. Pellagra was reported in more than thirty states in 1911. It caused 5 percent of the deaths at the Georgia State Sanitarium in 1908 and 20 percent in 1912. See *69th Annual Report of Georgia State Sanitarium* (1912), 26–27.

62. Edward W. Watson, "'Stern' Facts About Pellagra," *Medical Notes and Queries* 6 (April 1911): 42–43. Watson credits this vague statement to C. H. Lavinder, a doubtful attribution in view of Lavinder's stern reaction that same year to the attack on cottonseed oil.

63. George M. Niles, "Pellagraphobia: A Word of Caution," *JAMA* 58 (May 4, 1912): 1341; H. M. Green, "Report for the National Pellagra Commission," *Journal of the National Medical Association* 6 (1914): 1–3.

64. Niles, "Pellagraphobia"; *Baltimore* (Md.) *Sun,* February 6, 1910, and *Baltimore* (Md.) *News,* October 26, 1910, quoted in Notebook, Babcock Papers, Ch.

65. J. M. King, "Report on Pellagra at Nashville, Tennessee," *Tr., Natl. Conf.,* 171–179; Lavinder to Surgeon General, July 20, 1909, NA; "Abstract of Discussion," *JAMA* 63 (September 26, 1914): 1096–1097.

66. J. A. Albright to Babcock, September 7, 1911, Babcock Papers, SC; *Proceedings of Conference of State and Provincial Boards of Health, 1912* (Washington), 119.

67. *Records of the Proceedings Before Joint Committee To Investigate Georgia State Sanitarium* (Atlanta: Charles P. Byrd, State Printer, 1910), 151–152; *New York Times,* October 10, 1915, II, 17; *JAMA* 59 (November 23, 1912): 1917.

68. Charles J. Brim, "Job's Illness: Pellagra," *Archives of Dermatology and Syphilology* 45 (1942): 371–376.

69. Notebook, Babcock Papers, Ch.; "Abstract of Discussion," 1096–1097.

70. Niles, "Pellagraphobia," 1341–1342, his, "Present Status of the Treatment of Pellagra," *Tr., NASP,* 352–354, and his, "Treatment of Pellagra, An Optimistic Survey of its Present Status," *JAMA* 62 (January 24, 1914): 287.

71. Unidentified clippings, Babcock Papers, SC; *The State,* September 25, 1910.

72. *Atlanta* (Ga.) *Journal,* August 27, 1911; *Atlanta* (Ga.) *Constitution,* September 30, 1911; Milton M. Carrick, "What Everyone Should Know About Pellagra," unidentified clipping in Babcock Papers, Ch; J. Wright Nash to Congressman J. T. Johnson, August 14, 1911, NA; W. E. Lindsay to Johnson, August 14, 1911, NA; R. M. Grimm, "Pellagra: An Investigation of a Local Outbreak in Kentucky," *PHR* 26 (September 22, 1911): 1423.

73. H. D. Allen, Jr., "Mortality and Psychotic Illness," *SMJ* 33 (January 1940): 73; unidentified advertisement, NA; Bernard Wolfe, "Are Jews Immune to Pellagra?" *SMJ* 5 (March 1912): 116–124.

74. Deaderick and Thompson, *Endemic Diseases,* 387. Fowler's solution, named for an English physician, Thomas Fowler, is an alkaline aqueous solution of potassium arsenite.

75. Atoxyl and salvarsan are both trademarks for arsenic compounds that came into such popular use that they entered the language in uncapitalized form. Atoxyl is the trademark for the monosodium salt of p-arsanilic acid, sometimes used hypodermically in the treatment of syphilis. Salvarsan is the trademark applied to arsphenamine.

76. Deaderick and Thompson, *Endemic Diseases,* 387–388; E. H. Martin, "The Relative Value of Soamin and Salvarsan in the Specific Treatment of Pellagra," *Tr., NASP,* 369–375.

77. *69th Annual Report of the Georgia State Sanitarium* (1912), 26–27; W. J. Cranston, "Salvarsan in Pellagra," *JAMA* 58 (March 18, 1912): 1509–1510.

78. Clipping, n.d., *The Cleveland Medical Journal,* Babcock Papers, Ch; C. H. Lavinder, "Pellagra, Brief Comments on Our Present Knowledge of the Disease," *PHR* 28 (November 21, 1913): 2462–2463.

79. Charles T. Nesbitt to Surgeon General Rupert Blue, May 15, 1914, Charles T. Nesbitt Papers, Duke University Library, Durham, N.C.; Cranston, "Salvarsan in Pellagra," 1508–1509.

80. E. H. Bowling, "An Apparent Cure for Pellagra," *The American*

Journal of Clinical Medicine 17 (1910): 1288–1290; Isadore Dyer, "Some Differential Points in Skin Lesions of Pellagra," *Tr., Natl. Conf.,* 75–85; Ernest Palmer and William Lee Secor, "The Treatment of Pellagra by Autoserotherapy," *JAMA* 64 (May 8, 1915): 1566–1567.

81. H. P. Cole and Gilman J. Winthrop, "Transfusions in Pellagra," *Tr., Natl. Conf.,* 161–168; *Spartanburg* (S.C.) *Times-Democrat,* July 1, 1910, quoted in Notebook, Babcock Papers, Ch.

82. D. H. Yates, "The Treatment of Pellagra by Static Electricity," *Journal of Advanced Therapeutics* 33 (February 1915): 61–69, and his, "Pellagra Successfully Treated by Electricity," *American Journal of Electrotherapeutics and Radiology* 11 (1922): 217–219. A Texas physician also used electricity to treat pellagra. See J. W. Torbett, "The Diagnosis and Treatment of Pellagra," *The American Journal of Clinical Medicine and Surgery* 17 (1910): 1291–1293.

83. Rohrer, "Pellagra," 99; Niles, "The Present Status," 348–352; C. C. Bass, "Climatic Treatment of Pellagra," *JAMA* 55 (September 10, 1910): 940–941.

84. "Pellagracide and Ez-X-Ba," *JAMA* 53 (March 2, 1912): 648–649. A chemical analysis of Ez-X-Ba showed it to be an aqueous, slightly acid solution of ferric, aluminum, and magnesium sulphates with small amounts of alkalies and a slightly aromatic material extracted with ether.

85. Babcock, "Medico-Legal Relation," 395–401; *The* (Rock Hill, S.C.) *Evening Herald,* July 7, 1913.

86. For a discussion of this point, see L. B. Myers, "The Sociological Aspect of Pellagra," *Tr., NASP,* 407–409.

Chapter 2
Teamwork

1. C. H. Lavinder, Report to the Surgeon General, 1910, ms., Babcock Papers, Ch.

2. *The Literary Digest* 61 (October 29, 1910), 745.

3. Lavinder to Wyman, May 21, 1910, NA.

4. Pellagra Commission Report to Surgeon General, November 23, 1910, NA.

5. *Savannah* (Ga.) *Evening Press,* July 28, 1911; *Savannah Morning News,* August 5, 1911.

6. A. F. Lever to Wyman, August 26, 1911; NA; W. S. Rankin to John M. Faison, June 14, 1912, NA; *Wilson* (N.C.) *Times,* July 9, 1912;

Annual Report of Surgeon General, 1911, 14; *Proceedings of Conference of State and Provisional Boards of Health, 1912,* 121.

7. J. F. Siler and P. E. Garrison, *Pellagra, First Progress Report of the Thompson–McFadden Pellagra Commission* (New York: n.p., 1913), 3–4.

8. Jonathan Wright to Surgeon General Blue, March 8, 1912, Blue to Wright, March 14, 1914, NA.

9. Lavinder to Blue, July 9, 1912, NA; *Savannah Morning News,* June 9, 1911.

10. Lavinder to Kerr, August 11, 1911; Lavinder to Wyman, August 12, 21, 22, September 5, 1911; Lavinder to Blue, January 29, 1912; Blue to Lavinder, February 23, 1912: all Box 150, NA.

11. Lavinder to John Kerr, April 27, 1912, NA; Lavinder to Babcock, May 8, 11, 1912, Babcock Papers, SC.

12. Siler and Garrison, *First Progress Report,* 4; *Savannah Morning News,* June 9, 1911.

13. *Louisville* (Ky.) *Times,* August 23, 1911; Lavinder to Blue, February 2, 1912, NA.

14. Lavinder to Surgeon General, January 13, 1912, NA; Grimm to Doctor [Babcock?], May 5, 1912, Babcock Papers, SC.

15. Grimm to Wyman, October 1, 1911, NA; R. M. Grimm, "Pellagra, A Report on Its Epidemiology," *PHR* 28 (March 7, 1913): 427–450, (March 14, 1913): 491–513. Out of 995 cases, Grimm showed that 60.4 percent were white females, 25.3 percent white males, 10.2 percent black females, and 4.1 percent black males. Insanity occurred among 19 percent of the black male victims; 51 percent of the black female victims died. White women, aged twenty to forty, were affected more often than any other group.

16. *Annual Report of the Surgeon General, 1912,* 32.

17. Siler and Garrison, *First Progress Report,* 17–18; Siler to Babcock, May 13, July 6, 1912, Babcock Papers, SC; *The State* (Columbia, S.C.), May 9, 1912; *Spartanburg* (S.C.) *Herald,* editorial, August 1, 1921.

18. Siler and Garrison, *First Progress Report,* 5–26.

19. C. H. Lavinder, "The Association for the Study of Pellagra: A Report of the Second Triennial Meeting," *PHR* 27 (November 1, 1912): 1776; *The State,* October 4, 1912.

20. *Annual Report of Surgeon General, 1912,* 173.

21. *The State,* October 3, 6, 1912.

22. F. M. Sandwith, "Can Pellagra Be a Disease Due to Deficiency in Nutrition?" *Tr., NASP,* 97–98; J. G. Crowther, *Discoveries and*

Inventions of the 20th Century, 4th ed. (London: Routledge, 1955), 243–245. The spelling of tryptophane was later changed, the *e* being dropped; hereafter, the modern spelling will be used.

23. Copy of editorial on meeting of NASP, by Dr. Beverley R, Tucker, Richmond, Va., Babcock Papers, SC.

24. Casimir Funk, "Studies on Pellagra: The Influence of the Milling of Maize on the Chemical Composition and Nutritive Value of Meal," *Journal of Physiology* 47 (1913): 389–392. When it became evident that many of the accessory food factors were not amines, the *e* was dropped from vitamine; hereafter the modern spelling will be used.

25. Carl Alsberg to Babcock, October 23, 1912, Babcock Papers, SC. Funk wrote the United States Department of Agriculture in January 1914 requesting that samples of maize and hominy from the pellagra districts be sent to him for analysis. So far as can be determined, these samples were not sent. See Funk to USDA (marked "received January 30, 1914"), and R. M. Grimm to Funk, February 11, 1914, NA.

26. *Proceedings of Conference of State and Provincial Boards of Health in North America, 1912,* 116–117.

27. J. F. Siler, P. E. Garrison, and W. J. MacNeal, "Second Progress Report of the Thompson–McFadden Pellagra Commission," *Archives of Internal Medicine* 14 (1914): 289–293.

28. *New York Times,* September 1, 1913, 2, September 13, 1913, 20; "Pellagra Conference," *SMJ* 6 (September 1913): 690–691.

29. J. F. Siler, P. E. Garrison, and W. J. MacNeal, "A Statistical Study of the Relation of Pellagra to the Use of Certain Foods and to the Location of Domicile in Six Selected Industrial Communities," *Archives of Internal Medicine* 14 (1914): 294–373 passim.

30. *New York Times,* June 26, 1914, 22. Even the Thompson–McFadden Commission discarded the idea that pellagra was carried by the simulium fly, but popular magazines ran articles singling out this insect as the carrier. See "Another Fly to Swat," *The Literary Digest* 47 (November 22, 1913): 1003.

31. J. F. Siler, P. E. Garrison, and W. J. MacNeal, "The Relation of Methods of Disposal of Sewage to the Spread of Pellagra," *Archives of Internal Medicine* 14 (1914): 453–466; "Widening Pellagra Zone," *Scientific American Supplement* 78 (December 5, 1914): 359.

32. Herbert Montfort Morais, *The History of the Negro in Medicine,* vol. 1: *International Library of Negro Life and History* (New York: Publishers Co., Inc., 1969), 68, 87; H. M. Green, "Report for the National Pellagra Commission, *Journal of the National Medical Association* 6 (1914): 4–5.

33. "The Transmission of Pellagra by Means of Insects," *JAMA* 62 (March 24, 1914): 1020–1021.

34. Rupert Blue to Secretary of Treasury, July 16, 1913, NA.

35. C. H. Lavinder, "The Prevalence and Geographic Distribution of Pellagra in the United States," *PHR* 27 (December 13, 1912): 2076–2081, and his, "Pellagra, Prevalence and Distribution in Arkansas, Oklahoma, and Texas," *PHR* 28 (July 25, 1913): 1555–1558. Hayne's trouble in collecting statistics in South Carolina is typical. He twitted South Carolina doctors for ignoring the cards sent out by the state board of health for reporting the disease. Charleston doctors, he said, had reported only four cases, fifty of whom had since died.

36. C. H. Lavinder, "Pellagra in Mississippi," *PHR* 28 (October 3, 1913): 2035–2038.

37. Lavinder to Surgeon General, July 31, 1913, NA.

38. C. H. Lavinder et al., "Attempts To Transmit Pellagra to Monkeys," *JAMA* 63 (September 26, 1914): 1093–1094.

39. "Attempts to Produce Experimental Pellagra," *Scientific American* 105 (December 2, 1911): 490; Lavinder to John W. Trask, November 12, 1913, NA.

40. U.S., Congress, House, 63d Cong., 1st sess., 1913, Bill 6924.

41. Secretary of Treasury to W. C. Adamson, August 6, 1913, Rupert Blue to Secretary of Treasury, October 7, 1913, NA.

42. Tillman to Babcock, July 17, 1913, Babcock Papers, SC; *Spartanburg Herald,* August 1, 1921, September 21, 1930. After 1913, work of the Thompson–McFadden Commission was supported by Col. Robert M. Thompson and Dr. George N. Miller.

43. "Pellagra Spreading," *SMJ* 6 (July 1913): 481–482.

44. Memorandum for Secretary Relative to the Need of Hospital and Laboratory Facilities At Spartanburg, S.C., December 15, 1913, NA; W. G. McAdoo to Speaker of House, Dec. 30, 1913, 63rd Cong., 2d sess., Doc. 599.

45. *New York Times,* June 21, 1914, II, 5; J. F. Siler, P. E. Garrison, and W. J. MacNeal, "Relation of Pellagra to Location of Domicile in Spartan Mills, S.C., and the Adjacent District," *Archives of Internal Medicine* 20 (August 1917): 198–200. Before the Spartanburg site was selected, the Public Health Service was asked by individuals to locate the hospital in two other places, Madison, Fla., where electricity was the principal method used to treat pellagra, and Cleveland County, N.C., where the healing waters of Patterson Springs were credited with curing the disease.

46. Carl Voegtlin, memorandum, Dietary Studies Concerning the Etiology and Treatment of Pellagra, March 3, 1914, NA; Voegtlin to

Surgeon General, October 23, 1914, NA; Andrew Hunter, Maurice H. Givens, and Robert C. Lewis, *Preliminary Observations on Metabolism in Pellagra,* Hygienic Laboratory Bulletin 102 (1916), 39–67.

47. John T. Brantley to Walter Wyman, February 18, 1911, NA; *71st Annual Report of the Georgia State Sanitarium* (1914), 28–29.

48. *71st Report of Georgia Sanitarium,* 32–33; W. F. Lorenz, "Mental Manifestations of Pellagra," *PHR* 31 (February 4, 1916): 221–246.

49. Lavinder to Babcock, December 12, 1910, Babcock Papers, SC. Lavinder's and Babcock's book was the first large monograph on pellagra in the English language. Lavinder looked without success for a publisher in the North. The book was published by The State Company of Columbia, South Carolina. Babcock reported a great many copies were sold, and it received favorable reviews. See *The State,* January 9, 1911.

50. These were G. M. Niles, *Pellagra, An American Problem* (Philadelphia: W. B. Saunders Co., 1912), and Stewart R. Roberts, *Pellagra, History, Distribution, Diagnosis, Prognosis, Treatment and Etiology* (St. Louis: C. V. Mosby Co., 1913). Lavinder and Babcock dismissed Niles's work as "the first paraphrase of Marie" and Roberts' work as being backed by the "corn crowd." See Lavinder to Babcock, October 25, 1911, April 23, 1912, Babcock Papers, SC.

51. The Thompson–McFadden Commission suggested that apparent Negro immunity might be attributed to segregation. Negroes rarely came into contact with pellagrins, most of whom were white. See J. F. Siler, P. E. Garrison, and W. J. MacNeal, "The Incidence of Pellagra in Spartanburg, County, S.C., and the Relation of the Initial Attack to Race, Sex and Age," *Archives of Internal Medicine* 16 (1916): 209–210. The commission did not work in Mississippi where more Negroes than whites were affected.

Chapter 3
Meat, Meal, and Molasses:
An Indictment

1. Ralph C. Williams, *The United States Public Health Service, 1798–1950* (Washington: Commissioned Officers Association of the United States Public Health Service, 1951), 272; Rupert Blue to Goldberger, February 7, 1914, Joseph Goldberger Papers, University of North Carolina, Chapel Hill.

2. Goldberger (JG) to Mary Goldberger (MG), June 20, 1915, Goldberger Papers.

3. Members of the advisory board were William H. Welch, Johns Hopkins University, chairman; Simon Flexner, University of Pennsylvania; William T. Sedgwick, Massachusetts Institute of Technology; Victor C. Vaughan, University of Michigan; and Frank Westbrook, University of Minnesota.

4. Medical Officers Journal, Hygienic Laboratory, March 16, 1904, National Library of Medicine, Bethesda, Md. (NLM).

5. Blue to JG, February 7, 1914, Goldberger Papers.

6. JG to MG, February 9, 1914, Mary Goldberger, "Science Pigeon-holed," ms., Goldberger Papers. The most complete biography of Goldberger is Robert P. Parsons, *Trail to Light* (Indianapolis: Bobbs-Merrill, 1943). Shorter accounts are Robert Parsons, "The Adventurous Goldberger," *Annals of Medical History,* New Series 3 (1931): 534–539; T. Swan Harding, "Another Jew Without Money," *The Atlantic Monthly* 148 (August 1931): 166–170; Paul DeKruif, *Hunger Fighters* (New York: Harcourt Brace, 1928), 335–370; Louis Pelner, "Joseph Goldberger, MD, Benefactor of Mankind," *New York State Journal of Medicine* 69 (November 15, December 1, 1969): 2936–2941, 3050–3055; William H. Sebrell, "Joseph Goldberger," *Journal of Nutrition* 55 (1955): 3–12.

7. Rupert B. Vance, *Human Geography of the South* (Chapel Hill: University of North Carolina Press, 1935), 411–412.

8. Rupert Vance, *Human Factors in Cotton Culture* (Chapel Hill: University of North Carolina Press, 1929), 297. The fact that the frontier diet was more nutritious than the modern facsimile was demonstrated in 1929. Three communities high in the Blue Ridge mountains were studied intensively by sociologists. In one, people still lived in such primitive conditions that they had never seen a flag. The other two were slightly more advanced. Yet those who lived in the most primitive community had fewer nutritional deficiencies than those in the other two. They lived on whole corn, cabbage, dried apples, salt pork, occasional rabbits and squirrels, wild honey, and molasses. The sociologists observed that "food habits are part of a delicately balanced social complex. If one factor is changed, all others must be changed accordingly." See Mandel Sherman and Thomas R. Henry, *Hollow Folk* (New York: Thomas Y. Crowell Co., 1933), 42–44, 47–48.

9. Goldberger, "Memorandum on Pellagra," March 2, 1914, NA.

10. Joseph Goldberger, "The Etiology of Pellagra," *PHR* 29 (June 26, 1914): 1683–1686.

11. *Joint Committee To Investigate the State Sanitarium* (Atlanta: Charles P. Byrd, State Printer, 1910), 322–324, 509, 629. There is

no evidence that Goldberger ever saw this report. He did not refer to it.

12. Ibid., 256–262, 281.

13. Ibid., 629.

14. *70th Annual Report of the Georgia State Sanitarium* (1913), 24–25.

15. W. F. Lorenz, "The Treatment of Pellagra," *PHR* 29 (September 11, 1914): 2357–2358; W. F. Lorenz, "Mental Manifestations of Pellagra," *PHR* 31 (February 4, 1916): 241–242; Joseph Goldberger, C. H. Waring, and D. G. Willets, "The Prevention of Pellagra," *PHR* 30 (October 22, 1915): 3119–3124. Some of the white patients in Goldberger's ward had been given dietary treatment earlier by Dr. Y. A. Little of the hospital staff. Dr. Little subordinated his study so that Goldberger could care for the patients.

16. Joseph Goldberger, "The Cause and Prevention of Pellagra," *PHR* 29 (September 11, 1914): 2355–2356; JG to Surgeon General, September 21, 1914, NA. There are minor discrepancies in the actual number of cases of pellagra recorded at these orphanages. Goldberger cites 79 in the Methodist Orphanage and 130 in the Baptist Orphanage (both in Jackson) in "Prevention of Pellagra," 3120.

17. JG to MG, October 3, 1914, Goldberger Papers.

18. Goldberger et al., "Prevention of Pellagra," 3118–3119.

19. JG to Surgeon General, September 21, 1914, NA.

20. JG to MG, September 30, 1914, Goldberger Papers.

21. Ibid., October 5, 1914, Goldberger Papers.

22. Goldberger et al., "Prevention of Pellagra," 3120–3121; JG to MG, October 3, 1914, Goldberger Papers.

23. *Jackson* (Miss.) *Daily News,* September 9, October 13, 1914.

24. Report printed in *Jackson Daily News,* November 11, 1915.

25. Ibid., November 5, 1915.

26. JG to MG, June 26, 1914, Goldberger Papers.

27. Goldberger, "Cause and Prevention of Pellagra," 2356; J. Goldberger and D. G. Willets, "The Treatment and Prevention of Pellagra," *PHR* 29 (October 23, 1914): 2822–2825.

28. *Savannah* (Ga.) *Morning News,* October 26, 1914; *New York Times,* July 23, 1915, 18; Goldberger, "Cause and Prevention of Pellagra," 2356–2357.

29. Quoted in Goldberger et al., "Prevention of Pellagra," 3119. The italics are Roussel's.

30. JG to MG, September 17, 1914, Goldberger Papers.

31. David G. Willets to Dr. Jones, October 19, 1914, NA.

32. Goldberger et al., "Prevention of Pellagra," 3124–3125.

33. *72nd Annual Report, Georgia State Sanitarium, 1915,* 28–29. Many of the pellagra deaths at the institution occurred among the 267 patients who had the disease on admission. The superintendent noted that pellagrins were kept at home until they were in a state of delirium, too late for treatment to do much good. The situation was complicated by a state law that required ten days to elapse between the application for a lunacy hearing and the actual trial. Those who could not be cared for at home were housed in common jails and arrived at Milledgeville exhausted.

34. Ibid., 17.

35. JG to MG, June 20, 1915, Goldberger Papers; Goldberger et al., "Prevention of Pellagra," 3123.

36. JG to MG, November 29, 1914, Goldberger Papers.

37. *The State* (Columbia, S.C.), August 28, 1915.

38. H. W. Rice, "The Etiology of Pellagra in Children, A Study of Two Hundred Cases in Orphanages," *SMJ* 9 (1916): 778–785.

39. JG to MG, May 26, August, 3, 1916, Goldberger Papers.

40. Joseph Goldberger, C. H. Waring, and W. F. Tanner, "Pellagra Prevention by Diet Among Institutional Inmates," *PHR* 38 (October 12, 1923): 2364–2365.

41. Charles V. Chapin, *A Report on State Public Health Work* (Chicago: American Medical Association, 1915), cited by Francis Robbins Allen, "Public Health Work in the Southeast, 1872–1941: The Study of a Social Movement" (Ph.D. diss., The University of North Carolina, 1946), 347.

42. J. R. Ridlon, "Pellagra, Value of Dietary Treatment," *PHR* 31 (July 28, 1916): 1984–1988, 1996–1999.

43. G. A. Wheeler, "Treatment and Prevention of Pellagra by a Daily Supplemental Meal," *JAMA* 78 (April 1, 1922): 955–957. A total of 105 patients were treated in the outpatient clinic. All were white except 2. The all-Negro National Medical Association charged that whites were kept at the hospital for "treatment," but that Negroes were allowed only to come back and forth for food and advice. See H. M. Green, "Report of Pellagra Commission of National Medical Association," *Journal of the National Medical Association* 10 (1918): 163.

44. Carl Voegtlin to J. W. Kerr, October 9, 1915, NA.

45. Voegtlin to Surgeon General, October 23, 1914, NA. Voegtlin's hypothesis on the cause of pellagra is stated in his, "The Treatment of Pellagra," *JAMA* 63 (September 26, 1914): 1094–1096.

46. JG to M. J. Rosenau, January 7, 1915, JG to MG, January 23, 1915, Goldberger Papers. Rosenau, Goldberger's former superior at the Hygienic Laboratory, was by this time at the Harvard University Medical School.
47. JG to MG, April 25, 1915, Goldberger Papers.
48. *Savannah Morning News,* October 26, 1914, July 21, 1915. *The Jackson Daily* (Miss.) *News* reprinted the pamphlet in full, March 17, 1915.
49. JG to MG, June 20, 24, 1915, Goldberger Papers.
50. *The State,* November 17, 1914.
51. *Shreveport* (La.) *Times,* June 15, 1915; *New Orleans* (La.) *State,* July 17, 1915, clippings in Babcock Papers, SC.
52. JG to MG, November 29, 1914, Goldberger Papers.
53. JG to MG, December 19, 1914, July 24, August 19, 1915, Goldberger Papers; *New Orleans Times Picayune,* June 23, 1915, clipping in Babcock Papers, SC.
54. JG to MG, October 23, 1915, Goldberger Papers.
55. William S. Hall, "Psychiatrist, Humanitarian, and Scholar, James Woods Babcock, M.D.," *Journal of the South Carolina Medical Association* (October 1970): 370.
56. *The State,* October 21, 1915; program of Third Triennial Meeting in Babcock Papers, Ch. Transactions of the session were never published.
57. "Minutes of Third Triennial Meeting," ms., 88, Babcock Papers, SC; *The State,* October 23, 1915.
58. "Minutes," 111, Babcock Papers, SC.
59. *The State,* October 22, 1915.
60. JG to MG, October 23, 1915, Goldberger Papers.
61. "Minutes," 143–144, Babcock Papers, SC.
62. *The State,* October 22, 23, 1915.
63. Ibid., October 25, 1915.
64. *Report of the State Board of Health of Mississippi, 1913–1915,* 53; *1915–1917,* 101–102.
65. JG to MG, October 30, 1915, Goldberger Papers.
66. Joseph Goldberger and G. A. Wheeler, *Experimental Production of Pellagra in Human Subjects by Means of Diet,* Hygienic Laboratory Bulletin 120 (February 1920), 11–14. The first official report made of the prison experiment is Joseph Goldberger and G. A. Wheeler, "Experimental Pellagra in the Human Subject Brought About by a Restricted Diet," *PHR* 30 (November 12, 1915): 3336–3339.
67. Goldberger and Wheeler, *Experimental Production of Pellagra,* 7–11; *Jackson Daily News,* November 1, 2, 1915.

68. Goldberger and Wheeler, *Experimental Production of Pellagra,*
15–16.

69. Ibid., 18–23, 29–30.

70. Ibid., 48–92.

71. Ibid., 30–32. These were Dr. E. H. Galloway, secretary of the
Mississippi State Board of Health; Dr. Nolan Stewart, former superin-
tendent of the Mississippi Asylum for the Insane at Jackson; Dr. Marcus
Haase, professor of dermatology, Medical College of Tennessee,
Memphis; and Dr. Martin F. Engman, professor of dermatology, Wash-
ington University Medical School, St. Louis. The volunteers were also
seen by Dr. C. R. Stingily and Dr. F. C. Watkins of the Mississippi
State Board of Health and by Dr. C. H. Waring, assistant surgeon,
U.S. Public Health Service. Dr. Haase was a convert to the diet theory.
When he first met Goldberger in July 1914, he was a believer in
"infection" in pellagra.

72. JG to MG, October 30, 1915, Goldberger Papers. Goldberger
changed to six the number of men who had the skin rash in a letter
to his wife three days later. Six was the number used in the published
reports.

73. Ibid., November 2, 1915, Goldberger Papers.

74. *Jackson Daily News,* November 2, 1915; "The Puzzle of Pellagra,"
The Independent 84 (December 27, 1915): 505.

75. *Jackson Daily News,* November 1, 2, 1915.

76. JG to MG, October 30, 1915, Goldberger Papers.

Chapter 4
Praise and Protest

1. *Jackson* (Miss.) *Daily News,* November 1, 2, 1915; *The Clarion-
Ledger* (Jackson, Miss.), November 4, 1915; *New York World,* November 2, 1915.

2. JG to MG, August 25, October 29, 1915, Goldberger Papers.

3. Editorial, *Baltimore* (Md.) *Sun,* November 3, 1915; "Discussion:
Pellagra Symposium," SMJ 9 (1916): 35–37. The reaction of *The
State* (Columbia, S.C.), November 4, 1915, is interesting in view of
the fact that just two weeks earlier it had praised Goldberger's paper
at the National Association for the Study of Pellagra: "In view, however,
of former disappointments which have followed upon the first enthusiasm
of what have been claimed as facts by medical theorists and experi-
mentors we should keep our minds open till reports were in from

other observers, from other laboratories, from well controlled experiments and from many other countries in which pellagra is prevalent. The pellagra problem is too large to be solved off hand. Its solution requires patience, well-seasoned judgment, and above all time."

4. "Discussion: Pellagra Symposium," 31–42.

5. *The State,* November 12, 1915; "Discussion: Pellagra Symposium," 31–32.

6. "Discussion: Pellagra Symposium," 35–40.

7. Editorial, *Jackson Daily News,* November 12, 1915.

8. Paul De Kruif, *The Fight For Life* (New York: Harcourt Brace, 1938), 20–21.

9. Quoted in Soloman Kazan, "Joseph Goldberger," *Medical Record* 146 (1937): 476.

10. JG to MG, November 22 (?), 24, 1915, Goldberger Papers.

11. *Jackson Daily News,* November 17, 1915; unidentified clippings, Scrapbook 2, Goldberger Papers. The Tri-State meeting was attended by doctors from Mississippi, Arkansas, and Tennessee.

12. W. J. MacNeal, "The Alleged Production of Pellagra by an Unbalanced Diet," *JAMA* 61 (March 25, 1916): 975–977; Joseph Goldberger, "A Reply," *JAMA* 61 (March 25, 1916): 977.

13. William Deaderick and L. O. Thompson, *Endemic Diseases of the Southern States* (Philadelphia: W. B. Saunders Co., 1916), 301.

14. E. M. Perdue, *Pellagra* (Kansas City, Mo.: Burton Publishing Co., 1916), 343–344. Perdue was professor at the Eclectic Medical University in Kansas City and president of the American Association of Progressive Medicine. He claimed to be head of the largest laboratory in the world connected with pellagra research.

15. *Jackson Daily News,* November 12, 1915.

16. Carl Voegtlin to Director of Hygienic Laboratory, November 26, 1915, NA. Goldberger agreed to include references to Voegtlin's work in future publications. See A. M. Stimson to Voegtlin, December 3, 1915, NA. It is interesting to note that Voegtlin's outline of work for the Spartanburg hospital was submitted March 3, 1914, one day after Goldberger submitted his comprehensive plan for the entire pellagra study.

17. Francis Robbins Allen, "Public Health Work in the Southeast, 1872–1941: The Study of a Social Movement" (Ph.D. diss., University of North Carolina, 1946), 77–78, 111–112.

18. For a discussion of the reticence of Americans to accept Koch's ideas, see H. R. M. Landis, "The Reception of Koch's Discovery in the United States," *Annals of Medical History* 4 (1932): 531–537.

19. Elmer V. McCollum, *A History of Nutrition, Sequence of Ideas in Nutrition Investigation* (Boston: Houghton, Mifflin, 1957), 226.

20. Elmer V. McCollum, *From Kansas Farm Boy to Scientist* (Lawrence, Kan.: University of Kansas Press, 1964), 156–157.

21. E. Neige Todhunter, "Development of Knowledge in Nutrition: II, Human Experiments," 49, and E. V. McCollum, "An Adventure in Nutrition Investigation," 37, both in *Essays on History of Nutrition and Dietetics,* comp. Adelia M. Beeukes, E. Neige Todhunter, and Emma Seifrit Weigley (American Dietetic Association, 1967).

22. *Jackson Daily News,* November 2, 1915.

23. Nesbitt to Arthur W. Page, January 29, 1916, Charles T. Nesbitt Papers, Duke University Library, Durham, N.C.

24. Ibid.

25. Nesbitt to C. W. Stiles, April 21, 1916, Nesbitt Papers; JG to MG, January 14, 1916, Goldberger Papers.

26. Edward B. Vedder, "Dietary Deficiency as the Etiological Factor in Pellagra," *Archives of Internal Medicine* 18 (August 1916): 137–162.

27. Williams's interest in beriberi continued long after his work in the Philippines. In 1933 he finally isolated the antiberiberi factor, thiamine. He learned the structure of the molecule and was able to synthesize it by 1936.

28. Edward B. Vedder, *Beriberi* (New York: William Wood & Co., 1913), 317–318.

29. Oscar Dowling to doctors of Louisiana, June 2, 1915, NA; W. H. Sullivan to Edgar H. Farrar, November 10, 1915, Goldberger Papers; *36th Annual Report of the State Board of Health of South Carolina, 1915,* quoted in Roe Remington, "The Enigma of Pellagra," *SMJ* 37 (1944): 607; *The Jackson Daily News,* November 2, 16, 1915.

30. *Report of the State Board of Health of Mississippi, 1915–1917,* 101; *Jackson Daily News,* November 1, 1915.

31. F. L. Watkins, *A Statistical Report of Pellagra in Mississippi* (Jackson: Mississippi State Board of Health, 1915), 2–18, 28–33. To arrive at the cost, the average time lost from work was assumed to be six weeks at seventy-five cents a day. Cost of medicine was estimated at ten dollars a case, and funerals at twenty dollars each. There were 10,954 cases of pellagra in Mississippi in 1914, with 1,192 deaths.

32. Mississippi, *Laws of the State of Mississippi, 1916,* House Bill 820, 202.

33. Goldberger to Blue, September 12, 1918, NA.

34. Joseph Goldberger, "Pellagra, Its Nature and Prevention," *PHR* 33 (April 5, 1918): 487–488.

35. *Report of State Board of Health of Mississippi, 1915–1917,* 102.

36. "Cause and Cure of Pellagra," *Scientific American Supplement,* 81 (January 1, 1916): 11; William Petersen, "The Mortality from Pellagra in the Southern States," *JAMA* 69 (December 22, 1917): 2098. Peterson said the number of pellagra deaths in the South in 1915 was well over 10,000. This included, 2,012 in Georgia, an estimated figure since no statistics were collected in that state.

37. Goldberger, "Pellagra, Its Nature and Prevention," 483.

38. Joseph Goldberger, "The Transmissibility of Pellagra," *PHR* 31 (November 17, 1916): 3159–3162.

39. Medical Officers Journal, Hygienic Laboratory, June 7, 1916, NLM.

40. Goldberger, "Transmissibility of Pellagra," 3167.

41. JG to MG, June 25, 1916, Goldberger Papers.

42. Mary Goldberger, "Dr. Joseph Goldberger: His Wife's Recollections," *American Dietetic Association Journal* 32 (August 1956): 726; Goldberger, "Transmissibility of Pellagra," 3167.

43. *SMJ* 10 (1917), 383–390.

44. J. F. Siler, P. E. Garrison, and W. J. MacNeal, "Relation of Pellagra to Location of Domicile in Spartan Mills, S.C., and the Adjacent District," *Archives of Internal Medicine* 20 (August 1917): 258–259n.

45. Petersen, "Mortality from Pellagra," 2096.

46. H. M. Green, "Report of Pellagra Commission of N.M.A.," *Journal of the National Medical Association* 10 (1918): 164.

47. Henry F. Harris, *Pellagra* (New York: Macmillan Co., 1919), 115. Harris had difficulty finding a publisher. He wrote Babcock that Blakiston of Philadelphia had asked to publish the work, but as it grew in length, hard work, and expense, they got "cold feet," so Harris had assumed full responsibility for publishing the work himself. "The cost has been for one in my moderate circumstances very great, and now I am penalized for trying to do the thing as well as I know how. The really funny part of it is that they have all objected on the grounds that the work would be too complete!" Harris to Babcock, August 5, 1919, Babcock Papers, SC.

48. Harris, *Pellagra,* 9. It is interesting to note that the same year Harris's book appeared, several of Goldberger's articles on pellagra were being translated into Italian for distribution there. The translation was done at the suggestion of the American consulate in Naples.

49. Reid Hunt to JG, November 2, 1915; Allan J. McLaughlin to JG, December 6, 1915; E. V. McCollum to JG, January 1, 1917; JG to MG, December 4, 17, 1916: all Goldberger Papers.

Chapter 5
A Tale of Seven Villages

1. Goldberger and the Thompson–McFadden Commission agreed on only one point: those who used milk daily had little pellagra.

2. Joseph Goldberger, C. H. Waring, and D. G. Willets, "The Prevention of Pellagra," *PHR* 30 (October 22, 1915): 2128–2129; Joseph Goldberger, G. A. Wheeler, and Edgar Sydenstricker, "A Study of the Relation of Diet to Pellagra Incidence in Seven Textile-Mill Communities of South Carolina in 1916," *PHR* 35 (March 19, 1920): 654–655.

3. Goldberger et al., "A Study of Relation of Diet," 658–659.

4. Ibid., 660–663.

5. Ibid., 666–667. To insure uniformity, members of a household were considered in terms of adult male units. On this scale, devised by W. O. Atwood in 1915, an adult male was given a rating of 1, an adult female, 0.8, and the children, lesser numbers on a pro-rata basis according to age, or in the case of teen-agers, of age and sex.

6. Ibid., 669.

7. Ibid., 682–685, 690–693.

8. Joseph Goldberger, G. A. Wheeler and Edgar Sydenstricker, "Diet in Pellagra," *New York Medical Journal* 107 (June 15, 1918): 1146.

9. G. A. Wheeler, "Pellagra in Yancey County, North Carolina," *PHR* 35 (October 22, 1920): 2509–2513; Mathilde Koch and Carl Voegtlin, *Chemical Changes in the Central Nervous System as a Result of a Restricted Vegetable Diet*, Hygienic Laboratory Bulletin 103 (February 1916), 49.

10. Mrs. John Von Vorst and Marie Von Vorst, *The Woman Who Toils, Being the Experiences of Two Gentlewomen as Factory Girls* (New York: Doubleday Page & Co., 1905), 227, 234, 239.

11. Edgar Sydenstricker, "The Prevalence of Pellagra," *PHR* 30 (October 22, 1915): 3138–3141.

12. Carl Voegtlin, M. X. Sullivan, and C. N. Myers, "Bread As Food," *PHR* 31 (April 14, 1916): 935–943.

13. Ibid., 936–937. It was not then possible to isolate vitamins from natural foods, but a fairly accurate index to the relative amounts of vitamins present could be determined from the phosphorus content. Another indictment of modern milling methods was made a short time later by Dr. Edward Jenner Wood of Wilmington, North Carolina, who found no cases of pellagra in counties removed from the railroad

where waterground or whole grain cornmeal was still used exclusively. He said modern electric milling destroyed the protective substance. Unless users of this meal adapted their diet so that the vitamins thus destroyed were supplied in other foods, pellagra would follow. See *Scientific American Supplement* 82 (July 15, 1916): 43.

14. Voegtlin et al., "Bread As Food," 938–939, 942–943; *Report on Condition of Women and Child Wage Earners in the United States,* vol. 1, *Cotton Textile Industry* (Washington: Government Printing Office, 1910), 274.

15. William C. Edgar to Rupert Blue, telegram; *New York Globe,* quoted in John Lind to William G. McAdoo, April 27, 1916; William Crowder to Carl Alsberg, May 4, 1916: all NA. Dr. Wiley was architect of the Pure Food and Drug law of 1906.

16. *The Daily News* (Chicago, Ill.), July 14, 1916; *New York Times* September 8, 1917, 13.

17. Sydenstricker, "Prevalence of Pellagra," 3137; Carl A. Grote, "Pellagra: Diet as the Essential Element in Its Cause and Cure," *SMJ* 9 (1916): 229; Edward B. Vedder, "Dietary Deficiency as the Etiological Factor in Pellagra," *Archives of Internal Medicine* 18 (1916): 169; *The Atlanta* (Ga.) *Journal,* quoted in *The Union-Recorder* (Milledgeville, Ga.), March 30, 1915.

18. *Women and Child Wage Earners,* I, 502–504; Sydenstricker, "Prevalence of Pellagra," 3144; C. W. Stiles, "Diet and Pellagra," *PHR* 31 (March 31, 1916): 817–818.

19. Joseph Goldberger, G. A. Wheeler, Edgar Sydenstricker and W. I. King, *A Study of Endemic Pellagra in Some Cotton-Mill Villages of South Carolina,* Hygienic Laboratory Bulletin 153 (January 1929), 1, 66; Ralph C. Williams, *United States Public Health Service* (Washington: Commissioned Officers Association of the United States Public Health Service, 1951), 275; Goldberger to Blue, November 27, 1916, NA.

20. JG to MG, April 15, 1917, Goldberger Papers.

21. Ibid., March 25, 29, April 4, May 15, 20, 1917, Goldberger Papers.

22. Ibid., March 25, May 20, June 18, 23, 1917, Goldberger Papers. Goldberger saw so much of the disease that for the first time he showed some weariness in his work. He wrote his wife, September 23, 1917, "I'm very tired of it and feel the need of a mental rest from pellagra." His reference to Belgium was to the massive effort to prevent millions from starving there during World War I. The Commission for Relief in Belgium fed 10 million people during a four-year period.

23. JG to MG, July 1, 1917, Goldberger Papers; telephone interview with Dr. R. E. Dyer, one of the field investigators, in Atlanta, Ga., December 30, 1970.

24. JG to MG, July 1, 1917, Goldberger Papers. Goldberger invited Dr. Edsall to visit without first receiving approval from his Washington headquarters. Later he was worried lest Dr. Edsall's expenses should not be approved. "If . . . not, I am bankrupt!" he wrote his superior officer. To Goldberger's relief, the expenses were approved, notwithstanding the fact that the letter requesting approval came the day Edsall left Boston for South Carolina. See Goldberger to Kerr, July 2, 1917, NA.

25. David Edsall to Rupert Blue, July 23, 1917, NA.

26. Ibid.

27. Richard H. Follis, Jr., "Cellular Pathology and the Development of the Deficiency Disease Concept," *Bulletin of the History of Medicine* 34 (July–August 1960): 301–302; Burton J. Hendrick, "The Mastery of Pellagra," *The World's Work* 31 (April 1916): 639; Bess Furman Armstrong, "A Profile of the Public Health Service," ms., chap. 12, 32–33, NLM.

28. Two other nutrition authorities visited Goldberger at his work in Spartanburg and Milledgeville later in the year. They were Dr. William H. Welch of Baltimore and Dr. V. C. Vaughan, a member of the medical section of the Council of National Defense. Both agreed that pellagra was of dietary origin and that its eradication would be largely an economic problem. It could be accomplished only by securing for the people a properly balanced diet. V. C. Vaughan to Rupert Blue, December 27, 1917, W. H. Welch to Blue, January 14, 1918, NA.

29. Goldberger et al., *A Study of Endemic Pellagra,* 10–11; G. A. Wheeler, "A Note on the History of Pellagra in the United States," *PHR* 46 (September 18, 1931): 2226.

30. Goldberger et al., *A Study of Endemic Pellagra,* 11–12, 14–15.

31. Ibid., 13, 18.

32. Ibid., 33–37; JG to MG, August 14, 1917, Goldberger Papers.

33. *New York Times,* November 19, 1916, I, 6.

34. Joseph Goldberger, "The Relation of Diet to Poverty," *JAMA* 78 (June 3, 1922): 1679; Goldberger et al., *A Study of Endemic Pellagra,* 43; W. I. King, "Pellagra and Poverty," *The Survey* 46 (September 1, 1921): 631.

35. JG to MG, August 20, 1918, Goldberger Papers.

36. Sydenstricker, "Prevalence of Pellagra," 3134–3146.

37. *Report on Condition of Women and Child Wage Earners in the United States* (1910), 17 vols. Vols. 1 and 16 pertain to the cotton-mill industry.

38. See, for example, Kingsley Moses, "The Other Side of the Cotton Mill," *The Outlook* 113 (August 23, 1916): 977–984.

39. *The State,* October 27, 1915, May 3, 1916.

40. JG to MG, August 14, September 12, 1917, Goldberger Papers.

41. George Rosen, *A History of Public Health* (New York: MD Publications, Inc., 1958), 415; *New York Times,* May 14, 1917, 3.

42. Quoted in Maxcy Robson Dickson, *The Food Front in World War I* (Washington: American Council on Public Affairs, 1944), 75.

43. *The Spartanburg* (S.C.) *Journal,* March 31, 1917; *New York Times,* May 22, 1917.

44. Rupert P. Vance, *Human Factors in Cotton Culture* (Chapel Hill: University of North Carolina Press, 1929), 298–299.

45. Joseph Goldberger, G. A. Wheeler, and Edgar Sydenstricker, "A Study of the Relation of Family Income and Other Economic Factors to Pellagra Incidence in Seven Cotton-Mill Villages of South Carolina in 1916," *PHR* 35 (November 12, 1920): 2682–2684.

46. Ibid., 2686–2690. The figures cited were an incidence of 42.7 for incomes of less than $6 per adult male unit for a half-month period; 26.0 for the $6 to $7.99 group; 12.8 for the $8 to $9.99 group; 4.1 for the $10 to $13.99 bracket; and 3.4 for $14 and up.

47. Goldberger et al., "Relation of Family Income to Pellagra Incidence," 2693–2701. In this report, Inman Mills is referred to as "In" and Newry as "Ny."

48. Ibid., 2708–2709.

49. Ibid., 2709–2711.

50. *The State,* October 25, 1915.

51. King, "Pellagra and Poverty," 631–632.

52. Joseph Goldberger, "Pellagra, Its Nature and Prevention," *PHR* 33 (April 5, 1918): 484; Goldberger et al., *A Study of Endemic Pellagra,* 56–58; Goldberger to Dr. Schereschewsky, May 12, 1920, NA; Goldberger to Blue, June 8, 1920, NA.

53. *The Spartanburg Journal,* December 18, 1920.

54. Thomas C. Clark, *The Emerging South* (New York: Oxford University Press, 1961), 12–14.

55. Goldberger to Surgeon General Cumming, August 11, 1920, NA; JG to MG, July 28, 1920, Goldberger Papers.

56. Goldberger to Cumming, December 21, 1920, G. A. Wheeler to Cumming, February 1, March 7, 1921, NA.

Chapter 6
Famine, Plague, and Furor

1. Goldberger to Dr. Schereschewsky, July 9, 1921, NA.

2. W. S. Leathers to H. S. Cumming, July 18, 1921, NA.

3. Goldberger, "Memorandum Relative to Pellagra," July 18, 1921, NA.

4. *New York Times,* July 25, 1921, 1.

5. *The Spartanburg* (S.C.) *Herald* gave the story two paragraphs at the bottom of page one, July 23, 1921, while *The Spartanburg Journal* relegated it to two paragraphs on page 8 the same day. *The State,* Columbia's (S.C.) leading newspaper, did not use it at all.

6. Harding to Cumming, July 25, 1921, Harding to Farrand, July 25, 1921, Warren G. Harding Papers, Ohio Historical Society, Columbus, Ohio.

7. *Washington* (D.C.) *Star,* clipping, n.d., Scrapbook 2, Goldberger Papers; *New York Times,* July 26, 1921, 4.

8. "Outline of a Program for Dealing with Existing Pellagra Situation and Mitigating that Threatened for 1922," n.d., NA.

9. A. A. Coult to Surgeon General Cumming, July 26, 1921, NA; *Savannah* (Ga.) *Morning News,* July 28, 1921; R. B. Powell to Harding, July 27, 1921, Harding Papers.

10. Mrs. Roy W. McKinney to President Harding, July 26, 1921, Mrs. McKinney to Cumming, August 21, 1921, NA. Among those who pledged support for the PHS were the Columbia, S.C., Board of Health and the Texas Chamber of Commerce.

11. Harry Frank Farmer, "The Hookworm Eradication Program in the South, 1909–1925" (Ph.D. diss., University of Georgia, 1970), 2–4; *The State,* November 4, 1909.

12. *The State,* November 4, 1909; *Greensboro* (N.C.) *Daily News,* July 31, 1921.

13. Clipping, marked "Saginaw," July 29, 1921, Harding Papers.

14. Senator N. B. Dial to Surgeon General Cumming, July 18, 1921, NA.

15. *The State,* July 28, 30, 1921; *Congressional Record,* 67th Cong., 1st sess. (1921), 4430–4431.

16. James F. Byrnes to President Harding, July 27, 30, 1921, Harding Papers.

17. *Congressional Record,* 67th Cong., 1st sess. (1921), 4428, 4398, 4478, 4367.

18. Ibid., 4428.

19. Letter-to-editor, *The State,* clipping, n.d.; J. S. Wannamaker to Cumming, July 26, 1921; *Manufacturer's Record,* August 4, 1921, 75–77; all NA.

20. *New York Times,* July 27, 1921, 4; *The State,* July 27, 1921; North Carolina State Board of Health News Release, July 27, 1921, NA; unidentified clipping, Scrapbook 2, Goldberger Papers.

21. *Savannah Morning News,* July 27, 1921; *The Athens* (Ga.) *Banner,* July 30, 1921; *The Atlanta* (Ga.) *Constitution,* July 28, 1921; *New York Times,* July 27, 1921, 1, August 14, 1921, VI, 8.

22. *Memphis* (Tenn.) *Commercial Appeal,* quoted in *Congressional Record,* 67th Cong., 1st sess. (1921), 4457; *Birmingham* (Ala.) *News,* clipping, n.d., NA; W. O. Boger to Byrnes, July 27, 1921, Harding Papers.

23. *The Augusta* (Ga.) *Chronicle,* quoted in *New York Times,* July 27, 1921, 1; *Savannah Morning News,* July 28, August 5, 1921.

24. Miscellaneous letters, Box 154, NA.

25. Howard C. Smith to Harding, August 1, 1921, Harding Papers; *Greensboro Daily News,* August 2, 1921. Among the newspapers that took this stand were *The Macon* (Ga.) *News, Albany* (Ga.) *Herald, Dallas* (Tex.) *Morning News,* and *The Dallas Journal.*

26. Letter-to-editor, *The State,* clipping, n.d., NA; *New York Times,* July 28, 1921, 12; *Greensboro Daily News,* August 2, 1921.

27. *Spartanburg Journal,* August 2, 1921.

28. *Spartanburg Herald,* July 29, 1921.

29. George Tindall, *The Emergence of the New South, 1913–1945,* vol. 10, *A History of the South* (Baton Rouge: Louisiana State University Press, 1967), 123–124.

30. The Harris Laboratories to Harding, August 1, 1921; U.S. Food Products Corp. to Cumming, July 27, 1921; Celro-Salto-Nut Co. to PHS, August 11, 1921: all NA.

31. Thomas E. Wilson to Cumming, July 29, 1921; [Goldberger ?] to Norman Draper, August 8, 1921; H. S. Cumming to Borden Milk Co., August 6, 1921; Clarence J. Owens to Cumming, July 25, August 4, 1921: all NA.

32. *Minutes of Conference of State Health Officers of the South, August 4–5, 1921,* 3–10, 64–66, NA. Goldberger used census mortality figures for 1919 as the basis of his estimate. That year there were 2,806 deaths from pellagra recorded, but the registration area did not include Alabama, Arkansas, Georgia, Oklahoma, and Texas where the prevalence of the disease was known to be high. If these states had been included, he said, a conservative estimate of the number of pellagra deaths would

be 5,000. Since economic conditions were similar in 1920 to those of 1919, he used the same figure for that year. To be conservative, he reduced this by 20 percent to get a total of 4,000 deaths for 1920 from pellagra. Adding 25 percent for 1921, he got an estimated death rate for that year of 5,000. Since his surveys showed that not more than 5 percent of pellagrins died, he estimated the case rate at 100,000.

33. *Conference Minutes,* 19–25.

34. Ibid., 13–16, 27, 38–39, 56–59.

35. Ibid., 40–41, 53–54, 66, 101–102; "Resolutions of State Health Officers, August 5, 1921," NA.

36. Surgeon General Cumming to President Harding, August 9, 1921, NA. The minutes of the conference include only the notation that Dr. King spoke. The Surgeon General summarized his remarks in this letter to the President.

37. *Conference Minutes,* 88–89, 69–70.

38. Ibid., 79–81, 84–85.

39. Members of the committee were Dr. A. T. McCormack, Kentucky, chairman; Dr. C. W. Garrison, Arkansas; Dr. James A. Hayne, South Carolina; Dr. W. S. Leathers, Mississippi; and Dr. E. G. Williams, Virginia.

40. *Conference Minutes,* 58, 119; "Resolutions of State Health Officers"; *The Atlanta Constitution,* August 6, 1921.

41. Cumming to President Harding, August 9, 1921, NA. The department which Harding hoped to establish did not come into being for another thirty years, when the Department of Health, Education and Welfare was organized during the administration of President Dwight Eisenhower.

42. *Spartanburg Herald,* August 1, 17, 1921.

43. *The Spartanburg Journal,* August 23, 1921.

44. U.S., Department of Commerce, Bureau of the Census, *Mortality Statistics, 1921* (Washington: Government Printing Office, 1924), 67; Goldberger to Cumming, September 11, 1922, NA; Goldberger, "Report of Field Investigations of Pellagra for Fiscal Year, 1921–22," NA.

45. G. A. Wheeler to Mississippi State Board of Health, September 14, 1921, NA.

46. Ibid.

47. A. A. Coult to Senator Duncan Fletcher, August 20, 1921; Cumming to Senator Park Trammell, August 26, 1921; A. A. Coult to Cumming, August 31, 1921; Cong. W. J. Sears to Cumming, August 31, 1921: all NA.

48. *Spartanburg Herald,* August 30, 1921.

49. W. E. Deeks, "The Etiology and Treatment of Pellagra," *SMJ* 15 (November 1922): 891–898; "Discussion," *SMJ* 15 (November 1922): 899–905.

Chapter 7
The Quiet Search

1. JG to MG, September 23, 1921, Goldberger Papers.
2. Goldberger to Blue, December 20, 1917, W. H. Welch to Blue, January 14, 1918, NA.
3. Joseph Goldberger and W. F. Tanner, "A Study of the Pellagra-Preventive Action of Dried Beans, Casein, Dried Milk, and Brewers' Yeast with a Consideration of the Essential Preventive Factors Involved," *PHR* 40 (January 9, 1925): 54–55; *74th Annual Report, Georgia State Sanitarium, 1917,* 27. A second experiment using cowpeas conducted in the early 1920s was more successful in preventing pellagra, but this time the women were given more of the staple sanitarium diet of mush, rice, bread (both wheat and corn), and tomato juice. See Joseph Goldberger and G. A. Wheeler, "A Study of the Pellagra-Preventive Action of the Cowpea and Wheat Germ," *PHR* 42 (September 30, 1927): 2382–2387.
4. Joseph Goldberger and W. F. Tanner, "Amino-Acid Deficiency the Primary Etiological Factor in Pellagra," *PHR* 37 (March 3, 1922): 469–472; *Annual Report of Surgeon General, 1921,* 26–27.
5. Goldberger, "Report on Pellagra Field Investigations," July 15, 1921, Goldberger to Cumming, July 12, 1922, NA.
6. W. F. Tanner to Goldberger, August 5, 1921, quoted in R. C. Williams, *The United States Public Health Service, 1798–1950* (Washington: Commissioned Officers Association of the United States Public Health Service, 1951), 277. Goldberger was not the first to suggest the use of tryptophan for pellagra. The Surgeon General specified this as one of the projects which was to be carried out in July 1913. There is no evidence that this was done, however, before 1921.
7. Goldberger to Surgeon General, November 19, 1920, Goldberger to Dr. Schereschewsky, September 22, 1921, NA. Whether the last request for funds was granted cannot be ascertained. It probably was not since Goldberger referred to the treatment of only three patients with amino acids in his official report.
8. Goldberger and Tanner, "Amino-Acid Deficiency," 472–484; Joseph Goldberger and W. F. Tanner, "An Amino-Acid Deficiency

as the Primary Etiologic Factor in Pellagra," *JAMA* 79 (December 23, 1922): 2135.

9. Clifford Cooke Furnas, *Man, Bread and Destiny* (New York: Reynal and Hitchcock, 1937), 33–37. Magazines began to carry popular articles on nutrition. For example, one dealing specifically with pellagra and diet is Robert G. Skerrett, "Starving in the Midst of Plenty," *Scientific American* 125 (August 13, 1921): 116.

10. Elmer V. McCollum, *From Kansas Farm Boy to Scientist* (Lawrence, Kan.: University of Kansas Press, 1964), 114. A colorful account of Babcock's early work is given in Paul De Kruif, *Hunger Fighters* (New York: Harcourt, Brace, 1928), 267–297. De Kruif calls Babcock the "finder of the 'hidden hunger.' "

11. Joseph Goldberger and W. F. Tanner, "A Study of the Prevention and Treatment of Pellagra, Experiments Showing the Value of Fresh Meat and Milk, the Therapeutic Failure of Gelatin, and the Preventive Failure of Cod-Liver Oil," *PHR* 39 (January 18, 1924): 87–96.

12. Williams, *United States Public Health Service,* 183–194, 215–218, 246–248; Hygienic Laboratory Station Journal (1922), 5, NLM.

13. Joseph Goldberger and G. A. Wheeler, "Experimental Black-Tongue in Dogs and Its Relation to Pellagra," *PHR* 43 (January 27, 1928): 172–174. Chittenden and Frank P. Underhill of Yale University began their experimental feeding of dogs in 1905–1906. They noted that a diet of boiled peas, cracker meal, and cottonseed oil was positively injurious. In 1913, they repeated the experiment, feeding the dogs relatively large amounts of boiled peas and noted that larger quantities of peas delayed the onset of illness and extended the life span. In a later experiment, they gradually reduced the amount of meat fed to their test animals over a period of months. Even though there was always some meat in the diet, reduction in the quantity to an undefined limit caused death. Symptoms in all their test animals fed boiled peas, cracker meal, and salad oil resembled human pellagra. See Russell H. Chittenden and Frank P. Underhill, "The Production in Dogs of a Pathological Condition Which Closely Resembles Human Pellagra," *American Journal of Physiology* 44 (1917): 20, 28–29, 43–45.

14. G. A. Wheeler, Joseph Goldberger, and M. R. Blackstock, "On the Probable Identity of the Chittenden-Underhill Pellagra-like Syndrome in Dogs and 'Black-Tongue,' " *PHR* 37 (May 5, 1922): 1063–1069; Goldberger and Wheeler, "Experimental Black-Tongue in Dogs," 212.

15. Goldberger and Wheeler, "Experimental Black-Tongue in Dogs," 175–177.

16. Joseph Goldberger, G. A. Wheeler, R. D. Lillie, and L. M. Rogers, "A Study of the Black-Tongue Preventive Action of 16 Foodstuffs with Special Reference to the Identity of Black-Tongue of Dogs and Pellagra of Man," *PHR* 43 (June 8, 1928): 1385–1445; Joseph Goldberger, G. A. Wheeler, R. D. Lillie, and L. M. Rogers, "A Further Study of Experimental Black-Tongue with Special Reference to the Black-Tongue Preventive in Yeast," *PHR* 43 (March 23, 1928): 657–684; JG to MG, July 13, 1923, Goldberger Papers.

17. W. F. Tanner to Surgeon General, February 6, 1923, NA; Goldberger to Surgeon General, December 2, 1922, June 4, 1923, NA; Goldberger and Tanner, "Preventive Action of Dried Beans," 72.

18. Goldberger and Tanner, "Preventive Action of Dried Beans," 73–75. Actually, one patient who was given yeast died, but she was admitted to the hospital in such a debilitated condition that she lived only three days.

19. *New York Times,* March 31, 1925, 4; Folder 23, Goldberger Papers. The articles in *PHR* citing the value of yeast appeared in 40 (January 9, 1925): 54–80, and 40 (May 8, 1925): 927–28.

20. Goldberger and Tanner, "Preventive Action of Dried Beans," 72–73; J. Goldberger, G. A. Wheeler, R. D. Lillie and L. M. Rogers, "A Further Study of Butter, Fresh Beef, and Yeast as Pellagra Preventives," *PHR* 41 (February 19, 1926): 298–302.

21. J. Goldberger and G. A. Wheeler, "A Study of the Pellagra-Preventive Action of the Tomato, Carrot, and Rutabaga Turnip," *PHR* 42 (May 13, 1927): 1299–1306, their, "A Study of the Pellagra-Preventive Action of the Cowpea and Commercial Wheat Germ," *PHR* 42 (September 30, 1927): 2387–2390, and their, "A Study of the Pellagra-Preventive Action of Canned Salmon," *PHR* 44 (November 15, 1929): 2769–2770.

22. *82nd Annual Report of the Georgia State Sanitarium, 1925,* 24; *85th Report, 1928,* 25.

23. Goldberger et al., "A Further Study of Butter," 305–313; Joseph Goldberger and R. D. Lillie, "A Note on the Experimental Pellagra-like Condition in the Albino Rat," *PHR* 41 (May 28, 1926): 1025–1029; *New York Sun,* May 13, 1926; "Discussion," *SMJ* 21 (1928): 714; Joseph Goldberger, "Pellagra," *Journal of the American Dietetic Association* 4 (1929): 225. Several years after Goldberger's death, it was definitely proved that the pellagralike condition he had produced in rats was not the analog of human pellagra as he thought, but a condition produced by a deficiency of vitamin B_6, pyridoxine, something quite separate from P-P. See E. V. McCollum et al., *The Newer Knowledge of Nutrition,* 5th ed. (New York: The Macmillan Co., 1939), 506–507.

24. Folders 22, 23, 24, Goldberger Papers.

25. *Red Cross Courier* 6 (June 1, 1927): 7; *New York Times,* July 26, 1927, 33; Surgeon General to JG, July 23, 1927, Goldberger Papers; MG to JG, July 29, 1927, Goldberger Papers.

26. *The Mississippi Valley Flood Disaster of 1927, Official Report of Operations* (Washington: American National Red Cross, n.d.), 107–108; unidentified clipping, Scrapbook 2, Goldberger Papers.

27. *New York Times,* August 24, 1927, 39; Paul De Kruif, "The Rise and Fall of Pellagra," *Readers' Digest* 31 (September 1937): 76.

28. *Red Cross Courier* 6 (August 15, 1927), 4; (September 13, 1927), 6–7; (September 15, 1927), 29; (October 1, 1927), 14.

29. *Report of the State Board of Health of Mississippi, 1927–1929,* 201–202, 210, 87–88.

30. Joseph Goldberger and Edgar Sydenstricker, "Pellagra in the Mississippi Flood Area," *PHR* 42 (November 4, 1927): 2711.

31. *Annual Report of the Surgeon General, 1925,* 12.

32. De Kruif, *Hunger Fighters,* 362–363.

Chapter 8
A Practical Approach

1. Unidentified clipping, Scrapbook 2, Goldberger Papers; William DeKleine, "Recent Trends in Pellagra," *American Journal of Public Health* 27 (June 1937): 599; *Report of State Board of Health of Mississippi, 1927–1929,* 98; Dorothy Dickens, *A Nutrition Investigation of Negro Tenants in the Yazoo-Mississippi Delta,* Mississippi Experiment Station Bulletin 254 (1928); Paul S. Carley, "History of Pellagra in the United States," *The Urologic and Cutaneous Review* 59 (1945): 298.

2. C. W. Garrison, "The Economic Aspects of Pellagra," *SMJ* 21 (1928), 238.

3. Ibid., 237–238; "Discussion," *SMJ* 21 (1928): 240.

4. Goldberger, "Pellagra," *Journal of the American Dietetic Association* 4 (1929): 227. He addressed the association October 31, 1928.

5. Mary Goldberger, "Dr. Joseph Goldberger: His Wife's Recollections," *Journal of the American Dietetic Association* 32 (1956): 727. Numerous letters to Mrs. Goldberger after her husband's death, as well as newspaper clippings paying tribute to him, are found in the Goldberger Papers. The early newspaper accounts attributed Goldberger's

death to an unusual anemia not unlike pellagra. Mrs. Goldberger called this a "shocking misstatement of fact" and a "direct blow to all his years of research on pellagra." An autopsy showed that he died of hypernephroma of the left kidney.

6. J. Frank Wilson, "Arsphenamine in the Treatment of Pellagra," *SMJ* 23 (1930): reprint; G. A. Wheeler to Mrs. Goldberger, April 9, 1930, Goldberger Papers.

7. Sidney Bliss, "Considerations Leading to the View that Pellagra Is an Iron-Deficiency Disease," *Science* 72 (December 5, 1930): 577–578; "The Increasing Prevalence of Pellagra," *JAMA* 96 (February 21, 1931): 614; Wheeler to editor of *Science,* February 9, 1931, marked "letter not sent," USPHS General File, 1924–1935, No. 042532, NA (hereafter cited as NA File 2); Wheeler to Surgeon General, Feb. 26, 1931, NA File 2. Bliss's statement about molasses being poor in iron was disputed by Nellie Halliday of the Michigan Agricultural Experiment Station who pointed out that, on the contrary, molasses was a rich source of iron. Bliss replied that Southerners did not eat concentrated molasses, but syrup prepared on their own farms. See *Science* 74 (September 25, 1931): 312–313; 75 (March 4, 1932), 266.

8. "Treatment for Pellagra," *Science* 74 (December 18, 1931): Supplement 12; "Vitamins as Factors in Health and Food Values," *American Journal of Public Health* 19 (1929): 484–485; Beverley R. Tucker, "A New Conception of Pellagra," *Virginia Medical Monthly* 61 (1935): 686–690; G. W. McCoy to Surgeon General, December 28, 1931, NA File 2; C. E. Rice to R. C. Williams, n.d., NA File 2.

9. G. A. Wheeler, "The Prevention of Pellagra," *SMJ* 23 (1930): 302–303.

10. Josue de Castro, *The Geography of Hunger* (Boston: Little Brown and Co., 1952), 57, 93, 116–119.

11. Wheeler to W. F. Draper, November 17, 1930, NA File 2.

12. G. A. Wheeler, "The Pellagra-Preventive Value of Canned Spinach, Canned Turnip Greens, Mature Onions, and Canned Green Beans," *PHR* 46 (November 6, 1931): 2666–2668; G. A. Wheeler, "The Pellagra-Preventive Value of Autoclaved Dried Yeast, Canned Flaked Haddock, and Canned Green Peas," *PHR* 48 (January 20, 1933): 67–77; G. A. Wheeler, "The Pellagra-Preventive Value of Green Cabbage, Collards, Mustard Greens, and Kale," *PHR* 48 (June 30, 1933): 754–758; G. A. Wheeler and D. J. Hunt, "The Pellagra-Preventive Value of Green Onions, Lettuce Leaves, Pork Shoulder, and Peanut-Meal," *PHR* 49 (June 22, 1934): 732–736. In 1934, Dr. W. H. Sebrell prepared a list of foods rated good, fair, slight, and poor in relation

to their pellagra-prevention properties. It was widely used in institutions trying to wipe out pellagra while staying within their food budgets. See *PHR* 49 (June 29, 1934): 754–756.

13. DeKleine, "Recent Trends," 598; U.S., Department of Commerce, Bureau of the Census, *Mortality Statistics* (Washington: Government Printing Office, 1920–1930); Mary Ross, "Death Hits Back," *The Survey* 61 (February 15, 1929): 651–652.

14. DeKleine, "Recent Trends," 595–596; *Agricultural Outlook for Southern States, 1930–31,* USDA Miscellaneous Bulletin 102 (Washington: Government Printing Office, 1930), 47–48, 51.

15. James H. Rice to Bernard Baruch, March 31, 1926, James H. Rice Papers, Duke University Library, Durham, N.C.

16. *Spartanburg* (S.C.) *Journal,* July 8, 9, September 6, 1930; G. A. Wheeler and W. H. Sebrell, "The Control of Pellagra," *JAMA* 99 (July 9, 1932): 95–98.

17. "Southern Mill Villages, A Survey," *The American Federationist* 38 (September 1931): 1091–1093.

18. *The American Labor Banner,* September 20, 1930, clipping in NA.

19. *Spartanburg Herald,* September 20, 1930; Paul J. Smith, "Labor Day in Dixie in 1930," *American Federationist* 37 (1930): 1064–1067, 1330; *Gastonia* (N.C.) *Gazette* quoted in *Spartanburg Journal,* August 21, 1930.

20. *Relief Work in the Drought of 1930–31, Official Report of Operations of the American National Red Cross* (Washington: n.p., n.d.) 5, 7, 61, 73–74; DeKleine, "Recent Trends," 596–598. Relief work was directed by a Federal Drought Relief Committee headed by Dr. C. W. Warburton. Working with pellagra-control were three subcommittees composed of representatives from the USDA, the PHS, the Office of Education of the Department of Interior, and the Red Cross. These committees dealt with local programs, nutrition information, and food distribution.

21. *Relief Work in Drought of 1930–31,* 24–27; William DeKleine, "Control of Pellagra," *SMJ* 35 (1942), 994; "Decrease in Pellagra," *Science* 76 (December 16, 1922), Supplement 8.

22. *Relief Work in Drought of 1930–31,* 67–69; DeKleine, "Recent Trends," 596–597; Richard Osborn Cummings, *The American and His Food* (Chicago: The University of Chicago Press, 1940), 182.

23. DeKleine, "Control of Pellagra," 994, and his, "Recent Trends," 597–598.

24. *The Pineville* (Ky.) *Sun,* April 9, October 1, 1931.

25. Ibid., January 28, March 17, 1932.

26. Wheeler to Surgeon General, June 18, 1932, NA File 2. Whitley County, Kentucky, launched a pellagra-control program that year. It was financed by a grant of $3,500 from American Women's Hospitals, New York, and by appropriations of $2,500 from the state and $500 from the county. See *JAMA* 98 (February 6, 1932): 486.

27. Wheeler to Surgeon General, January 19, 1933, NA File 2.

28. Francis Robbins Allen, "Public Health Work in the Southeast, 1872–1941: The Study of a Social Movement" (Ph.D. diss., University of North Carolina, 1946), 355; "Vitamins as Factors," 486; *Spartanburg Herald,* September 21, 1930.

29. Susan J. Mathews, *Food Habits of Georgia Rural People,* Georgia Experiment Station Bulletin 159 (1919), 15–17.

30. Madge Cheshire Vaughan, "Pellagra in Lee County, South Carolina: Its Physical, Economic, and Social Causes and Effects" (Master's thesis, University of South Carolina, 1933), 48, 40.

31. Hazel K. Stiebeling and Hazel Munsell, *Food Supply and Pellagra Incidence,* USDA Technical Bulletin 333 (Washington: Government Printing Office, 1931), 2–3, 15–20, 29.

32. T. J. Woofter, *Landlord and Tenant on the Cotton Plantation,* WPA Research Monograph 5 (Washington: Government Printing Office, 1936), 102; "Vitamins as Factors in Health," 486.

33. Hazel K. Stiebeling and Miriam Birdseye, *Adequate Diets for Families with Limited Incomes,* USDA Miscellaneous Publication 113 (Washington: Government Printing Office, 1931), 7–8; G. W. McCoy, memorandum, January 8, 1931, NA File 2; W. H. Sebrell to Assistant Surgeon General L. R. Thompson, December 8, 1933, NA File 2; *Standard Education Almanac 1969* (Los Angeles: Academic Media, Inc., 1969), 465.

34. *New York Times,* July 31, 1927, VIII, 10, March 18, 1929, 25, May 10, 1929, 29; Frederick D. Mott and Milton I. Roemer, *Rural Health and Medical Care* (New York: McGraw-Hill Book Co., 1948), 111.

35. DeKleine, "Control of Pellagra," 992–994; Bureau of the Census, *Mortality Statistics,* 1925, 1935, 1940. The number of deaths from pellagra in the United States in 1925 was 3,344; in 1935, 3,543; in 1940, 2,123.

36. Cummings, *The American and His Food,* 181; Joseph Gillman and Theodore Gillman, *Perspectives in Human Nutrition* (New York: Grune and Stratton, 1951), 59; Ira Robinson and Francis J. Clune, Jr., "Nutritional Disease, Culture, and Social Change," ms., in files

of the author. Yeast was distributed by the State Health Department of Georgia until 1962.

37. C. J. Milling, "Pellagra and the New Deal," *Journal of the South Carolina Medical Association* 32 (1936): 209–213; DeKleine, "Control of Pellagra," 994–995; Cummings, *The American and His Food,* 182, 188–189. DeKleine did not think food relief programs had much effect on the problem of pellagra. He claimed that the free distribution of food did little to alter the dietary habits of the people.

38. Wilma Dykeman and James Stokeley, *Seeds of Southern Change, The Life of Will Alexander* (Chicago: University of Chicago Press, 1962), 235–237.

39. Paul De Kruif, *The Fight for Life* (New York: Harcourt Brace, 1938), 23–26.

Chapter 9
Victory

1. C. A. Elvehjem, R. J. Madden, F. M. Strong, D. W. Wooley, "Relation of Nicotinic Acid and Nicotinic Acid Amide to Canine Black Tongue," *Journal of American Chemical Society* 59 (1937): 1767–1768; C. J. Koehn, Jr., and C. A. Elvehjem, "Further Studies on the Concentration of the Antipellagra Factor," *Journal of Biological Chemistry* 118 (1937): 693–699.

2. C. A. Elvehjem, "A Forty-Year Look at Nutrition Research," in *Essays on History of Nutrition and Dietetics,* comp. Adelia Beeukes, E. Neige Todhunter, and Emma Seifrit Weigley (Chicago: American Dietetic Association, 1967), 54–55.

3. "Nicotinic Acid and Pellagra," *SMJ* 31 (1938): 33; *Science News Letter* 34 (November 19, 1938): 323. Among those contributing to the fund were physicist Dr. Albert Einstein and Dr. Harold C. Urey, discoverer of heavy hydrogen.

4. C. A. Elvehjem, "Relation of Nicotinic Acid to Pellagra," *Physiological Reviews* 20 (1940), 260; *The Notifiable Diseases, Prevalence in States, 1940,* Supplement 166 to PHR 3; *The Notifiable Diseases, Prevalence in States, 1945,* Supplement 193 to PHR 9; *The Commonweal* 29 (November 4, 1938), 33. There were probably more cases of the disease than these figures show. Only twenty-one states reported case figures in these years, and some of these could not have been complete. In 1943, for example, Mississippi reported 2,748 cases with 84 deaths, while Georgia reported only 208 cases with 175 deaths. It is doubtful

that the disease was so much more fatal in Georgia; it is more probable that several thousand cases in Georgia were not reported at all. See *Notifiable Diseases, 1943,* Supplement 182 to *PHR.*

5. Sir John Boyd Orr, *Food, Health and Income, Report on a Survey of Diet in Relation to Income,* 2d. ed. (London: Macmillan, 1936), 56.

6. *Final Report of the Mixed Committee on the League of Nations on the Relations of Nutrition to Health, Agriculture and Economic Policy* (Geneva: Public Report of League of Nations, 1937), 31–37.

7. André Mayer, *Nutrition and Society,* World Food Publications No. 1 (Rome: Food and Agricultural Organization of the United Nations, 1956), 7–9.

8. Ibid., 14–15.

9. *New York Times,* January 22, 1941, 1, June 9, 1942, 20; V. P. Sydenstricker, "History of Pellagra," *American Journal of Clinical Nutrition* 6 (1958), 413–414.

10. E. V. McCollum, "From Hopkins to the Present," in *Essays on Nutrition and Dietetics,* 121–122.

11. Edward H. Beardsley, *Harry L. Russell and Agricultural Science in Wisconsin* (Madison: The University of Wisconsin Press, 1969), 148, 155–165 passim.

12. National Academy of Sciences, National Research Council, *Enrichment of Flour and Bread, A History of the Movement,* Bulletin 110 (Washington: National Academy of Sciences, 1944), 1–3; Russell M. Wilder, "A Brief History of the Enrichment of Bread and Flour," *JAMA* 162 (December 22, 1956): 1539–1540.

13. Wilder, "A Brief History," 1540; *New York Times,* January 10, 1941, 9; National Academy of Sciences, *Enrichment of Flour and Bread,* 4–5.

14. *New York Times,* January 12, 1941, IV, 8, January 30, 1941, 14.

15. *Proceedings of the National Nutrition Conference for Defense* (Washington: Government Printing Office, 1942), 1–2, 6, 221.

16. Ibid., ix, 220–221, 232.

17. Lydia J. Roberts, "Beginnings of the Recommended Dietary Allowances," in *Essays on Nutrition and Dietetics,* 110.

18. H. E. Jacob, "Bread in the Twentieth Century," *Ciba Symposia* 8 (1946): 493; Wilder, "A Brief History," 1540. South Carolina was also among the first to require by law that cornmeal be enriched. Alabama and Mississippi soon followed suit, an important step toward eradicating pellagra.

19. National Academy of Sciences, *Enrichment of Flour and Bread,* 48–49, 53–54.

20. Jane Stafford, "Decrease in Pellagra and Beriberi," *Science* 98 (July 30, 1943): Supplement 8; *New York Times,* November 15, 1942, IV, 11.

21. National Academy of Sciences, *Enrichment of Flour and Bread,* 45–46.

22. Margaret T. Cussler and Mary L. DeGive, "Outline of Studies on Food Habits in Rural Southeast," *The Problem of Changing Food Habits,* National Research Council Bulletin 108 (Washington: National Academy of Sciences, 1943), 109–112.

23. W. A. Krehl, L. J. Tepley, and C. A. Elvehjem, "Effect of Corn Grits on Nicotinic Acid Requirements of the Dog," *Proceedings, Society for Experimental Biology and Medicine* 58 (April 1945): 336–337. The authors said that the nicotinic acid content of grits should be increased to five times the unenriched level. They also found that white corn retarded the growth of experimental animals more than yellow corn. White corn is preferred to yellow in the South for grits and meal. See Krehl, Tepley, and Elvehjem, "Corn as an Etiological Factor in Production of a Nicotinic Acid Deficiency in the Rat," *Science* 101 (March 16, 1945): 283. Work on the relationship of corn to pellagra was conducted at other universities as well, notably at Auburn University in Alabama.

Too late for inclusion in the text, Professor Kenneth Carpenter of the University of Cambridge called to the author's attention another intriguing connection of maize consumption and pellagra. In a letter to the author, February 29, 1972, he wrote, "Wherever maize has been used by poor people as their staple food, without much meat or milk, there has been pellagra *except* in the traditional maize-eating area of Central America. When maize was taken from there around the world, the traditional cooking procedure was not followed. This, of course, includes a preliminary period of soaking in alkaline lime water. . . . There is evidence now that the niacin in maize (*and* other grains) is nutritionally unavailable, unless it has been treated with either acid or alkali. This appears to explain the observation that lime-treated tortillas will support the growth of rats where ordinary maize does not (unless free niacin is added.) If this train of argument is correct, then the poor in Europe and the Southern U.S.A. *could* have remained free of pellagra if they had adopted the cooking method of the Central Americans along with their crop."

24. W. A. Krehl, L. J. Tepley, P. S. Sarma, and C. A. Elvehjem,

"Growth-Retarding Effect of Corn in Nicotinic Acid-Low Ration and Its Counteraction by Tryptophan," *Science* 101 (May 11, 1945), 490; R. C. Williams, *The United States Public Health Service, 1798–1950* (Washington: Commissioned Officers Association of the United States Public Health Service, 1951), 277–278. Further research showed that the metabolism of tryptophan depended on the B vitamins, pyridoxine and riboflavin. Pyridoxine is essential for the synthesis of niacin from amino acid. See V. P. Sydenstricker, "The History of Pellagra, Its Recognition as a Disorder of Nutrition and Its Conquest," *American Journal of Clinical Nutrition* 6 (1958): 409–414.

A Note

on Sources

THE LITERATURE ON PELLAGRA is voluminous. Thousands of articles and a number of books written on the subject in English since the disease first appeared in the United States in the early part of this century have added to the already large volume of material from the eighteenth and nineteenth centuries, found especially in French, Spanish, and Italian journals. Since this study is confined to an analysis of the disease in the American South, particularly its social and economic aspects, it is based largely on twentieth century sources.

Manuscript collections are the most useful. The role of the United States Public Health Service in unraveling the etiology of pellagra is found in the *Joseph Goldberger Papers* in the Southern Historical Collection at the University of North Carolina, Chapel Hill, and in the *General Files of the United States Public Health Service* in the National Archives, Washington, D.C. (File 1648 dealing with material from 1897 to 1923 and File 0425-32 dealing with the years 1924 to 1935). The most valuable source for study of the early history of pellagra is the *James Woods Babcock Papers* in the South Caroliniana Library, Columbia, South Carolina. These papers are uncataloged and have not been used previously. Particularly useful are this collection's large number of newspaper clippings. A smaller collection of *James Woods Babcock Papers* is found in the Library of the Medical University of South Carolina at Charleston. These also are uncataloged.

The *Warren G. Harding Papers,* available on microfilm from the Ohio Historical Society, Columbus, contain some material on the President's role in the furor over pellagra in the summer of 1921. Two manuscript collections at Duke University, Durham, North Carolina, the *Charles T. Nesbitt Papers* and the *James H. Rice Collection,* contain some relevant materials.

The most readily available sources for studying the early ideas on the cause and cure of pellagra in the United States are the *Transactions of the National Conference on Pellagra* (Columbia, S.C.: The State Co., Printers, 1910), and *Transactions of the National Association for the Study of Pellagra* (Columbia, S.C.: The R. L. Bryan Co., 1914). *Public Health Reports* also printed numerous articles on pellagra after 1908, the most important of the early articles being written by Claude H. Lavinder and R. M. Grimm. Work of the Thompson–McFadden Commission was published in *Pellagra, First Progress Report of the Thompson–McFadden Pellagra Commission of the New York Post-Graduate School and Hospital* (New York: n.p., 1914). Subsequent reports of this commission were published in *Archives of Internal Medicine,* vol. 14 (1914), vol. 18 (1916), and vol. 20 (1917).

The most important work done on pellagra was that of Dr. Joseph Goldberger. The many articles he wrote on the disease, both alone and in collaboration with others, primarily are found scattered in *Public Health Reports,* volumes 29 (1914) through 44 (1929) and in the *Hygienic Laboratory Bulletins* (Washington: Government Printing Office), nos. 120 and 153 being particularly useful. A convenient collection of the most important of these papers, with a thoughtful essay on Goldberger's work by Milton Terris, is *Goldberger on Pellagra* (Baton Rouge: Louisiana State University Press, 1964). The most complete biography of Goldberger is Robert Percival, *Trail to Light: A Biography of Joseph Goldberger* (Indianapolis: Bobbs-Merrill, 1943). A shorter study of Goldberger's work on pellagra is included in *Hunger Fighters* by Paul De Kruif (New York: Harcourt Brace, 1928), written after several personal interviews with Goldberger late in the doctor's life.

Providing background on the varied functions of the Public Health Service during the period embraced in this study is *The United States Public Health Service, 1798–1950* by Ralph Chester Williams (Washington: Commissioned Officers Association of the United States Public Health Service, 1951). Also useful is an unpublished manuscript by Bess Furman Armstrong, "A Profile of the Public Health Service," a copy of which is in the National Library of Medicine at Bethesda, Maryland. Also at the NLM is the manuscript copy of the *Medical*

Officers Journal of the Hygienic Laboratory, which provides some personal insight into work of the laboratory during those years when Goldberger was on the staff.

Much of the controversy over pellagra may be traced in the pages of the *Southern Medical Journal,* beginning as early as vol. 2 (1909) and increasing in intensity after Goldberger began his work in 1914. For years papers on pellagra were presented at nearly every meeting of the Southern Medical Association, and the *SMJ* printed these, as well as transcriptions of the discussions which followed. The long debate over pellagra may also be followed in the *Journal of the American Medical Association.*

Useful for understanding the development of the peculiar pattern of Southern agriculture are several books by Rupert B. Vance; *Human Geography of the South,* 2d ed. (Chapel Hill: University of North Carolina Press, 1935), *Human Factors in Cotton Culture* (Chapel Hill: University of North Carolina Press, 1929), and *Farmers Without Land* (New York: Public Affairs Committee Pamphlet #12, 1937). Also valuable are George B. Tindall, *The Emergence of the New South, 1913–1945* (Baton Rouge: Louisiana State University Press, 1969), and Thomas D. Clark, *The Emerging South* (New York: Oxford University Press, 1961). Important for understanding the impact of the New Deal on pellagra is *Seeds of Southern Change: The Life of Will Alexander* by Wilma Dykeman and James Stokeley (Chicago: University of Chicago Press, 1962).

Works on the history of nutrition are too numerous to be cited here. However, those dealing with pioneer work at the University of Wisconsin particularly germane to the study of pellagra are Wilbur H. Glover, *Farm and College: The College of Agriculture at the University of Wisconsin. A History* (Madison: The University of Wisconsin Press, 1952); Elmer V. McCollum, *From Kansas Farm Boy to Scientist* (Lawrence: University of Kansas Press, 1964); and Edward H. Beardsley, *Harry L. Russell and Agricultural Science in Wisconsin* (Madison: University of Wisconsin Press, 1969.) Among the more valuable works on the history of nutrition is E. V. McCollum, *A History of Nutrition, The Sequence of Ideas in Nutrition Investigations* (Boston: Houghton-Mifflin, 1957).

Discovery of nicotinic acid as the pellagra-preventive vitamin was made at the University of Wisconsin and was reported by C. A. Elvehjem, R. J. Madden, F. M. Strong, and D. W. Wooley in the *Journal of American Chemical Society* 59 (1937): 1767–1768. An important article, "Relation of Nicotinic Acid to Pellagra" by Elvehjem was published in *Physiological Reviews* 20 (1940), 249–271. Among staff members at the Public Health Service who followed up Goldberger's work is W. H. Sebrell, who gives a summary of the work through the 1960s in "Clinical Nutrition in the United States," *American Journal of Public Health* 58 (1968): 2035–2042.

Newspaper files provide information on the social aspects of pellagra available no place else. Especially valuable is the *New York Times.* Southern newspapers which are rich sources are *The* (Columbia, South Carolina) *State, The Spartanburg* (South Carolina) *Herald* and *The Spartanburg Journal,* and *The Jackson* (Mississippi) *Daily News.* The South Carolina papers are useful for this study from about 1909 through 1921; the Mississippi paper is particularly useful for 1914 and 1915. The *New York Times,* indexed since 1913, includes some items on pellagra throughout the entire period of this study. A large number of newspaper clippings found in both collections of the *James Woods Babcock Papers,* the *Joseph Goldberger Papers,* the *Warren G. Harding Papers,* and in the pellagra file at the National Archives are also useful.

The most complete account of the addition of synthetic vitamins to bread and flour during World War II, which did much to reduce the incidence of pellagra and beriberi and other nutritional diseases in the United States, is *Enrichment of Flour and Bread, A History of the Movement* (Washington: National Academy of Science Bulletin No. 110, 1944). A shorter account is Russell M. Wilder, "Brief History of the Enrichment of Bread and Flour," *Journal of the American Medical Association* 162 (December 22, 1956): 2539–2541.

Recent accounts of the continuing battle against hunger in America are Senator Ernest F. Hollings *The Case Against Hunger: A Demand for a National Policy* (New York: Cowles Book Co., Inc., 1970), and Nick Kotz, *Let Them Eat Promises: The Politics of Hunger in America* (Englewood Cliffs, N.J.: Prentice-Hall, 1969).

Index